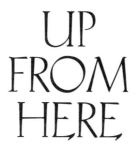

UP
FROM
HERE

UP FROM HERE

Reclaiming the Male Spirit:
A Guide to Transforming Emotions
into Power and Freedom

Iyanla Vanzant

HarperSanFrancisco
A Division of HarperCollins*Publishers*

HarperCollins books may be purchased for educational, business, or sales promotional use. For information please write: Special Markets Department, HarperCollins Publishers, Inc., 10 East 53rd Street, New York, NY 10022. HarperCollins Web site: http://www.harpercollins.com

HarperCollins®, ■®, and HarperSanFrancisco™ are
trademarks of HarperCollins Publishers, Inc.

FIRST EDITION
Designed by Joseph Rutt

Library of Congress Cataloging-in-Publication Data
Vanzant, Iyanla.
Up from here : reclaiming the male spirit : a guide to transforming emotions
into power and freedom / Iyanla Vanzant. — 1st ed.
p. cm.
Includes index
ISBN 0–06–251759–7 (alk. paper)
1. Men—Psychology. 2. Men—Conduct of life. 3. Emotions.
4. Self-actualization (Psychology). I. Title.
HQ1090.V345 2002
305.31—dc21
2002190209

02 03 04 05 06 ❖ QUE 10 9 8 7 6 5 4 3 2 1

This book is dedicated to Oluwalomoju Adeyemi Vanzant, Adesola Lewis Vanzant, and David Vanzant, my grandsons; Johnathan Harris, my nephew; and all of my fathers, brothers, sons, and grandsons currently serving time in God's Vacation Retreat Centers, also known as prisons.

May the power and force of your authentic identity guide you through the challenges of being human while awakening your hearts to the unlimited possibilities of your spiritual nature.

Contents

Introduction   1

1   Up from Here   13

2   Roy
Speaking Up   30

3   Phillip
Acting Up and Acting Out   75

4   Eddie
Building Spiritual Muscle   108

5   Gabriel
Not All Men Are Macho   133

Contents

6   Martin
    Taking Care of Unfinished Business   153

7   Garen
    What Makes a Man   172

8   Henry
    Overcoming Feelings of Inadequacy   194

    Epilogue   211

    Acknowledgments   215

    Index   217

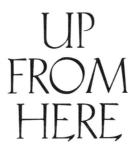

UP
FROM
HERE

Introduction

This book began on a morning drive to work. The thought
hit me like a ton of bricks: "Terror will kill you!" I had
been thinking about a young man I knew who had been mur-
dered. Shot in the head, at point-blank range, by someone he
knew. Someone named "Terror." You would think that if you
met a person whose name was Terror, you would run in
another direction. If, on the other hand, you are a young man
who feels somewhat lost, misplaced, and rather hopeless, it is
understandable that you would allow terror into your life. In
fact, it is understandable that terror would control your life.
Against everyone's warnings and pleading, this young man
started keeping company with Terror. Before long, Terror
had complete control of this young man's mind. He allowed

Terror to coerce him into doing things he knew he had no business doing. This young man wanted so much to belong, to have a place, to feel and be important, he could not see that terror would soon stop him dead in his tracks. For most men, terror does just that. Men are often terrorized by thoughts of failure, thoughts of not measuring up. In response to the terror they feel in their hearts, they will often brutalize themselves. They become driven. In some cases, men whose minds and hearts are filled with terror will brutalize those around them. In this case, where Terror had a face and two legs, terror didn't just brutalize a beautiful young man I had watched grow up before my eyes; it robbed him of his life.

Thinking about him that morning on my way to work, I realized I had left unfinished the work I had begun in 1993 with a book called *The Spirit of a Man: A Vision of Transformation for Black Men and the Women Who Love Them.* I wrote that book to say simply and plainly what people had been unable or afraid to say: God loves you men. He loves each one of you, not because you're Black, or because you're White, or because you're Asian, or because you're male. He loves you because you're made in his image and likeness. You're a part of God. Because you don't realize this, you're dying. And as you die, you take a vital piece of God's love and beauty with you. As a healer, I just couldn't leave that situation untended.

I realized that sunny morning on the bridge that I had to continue to write to you—to *all* men (and to all the women in your lives)—because you're continuing to die, not just on the battlefield, but inside, in your spirit. The world needs your light. The world needs your life. Every woman and child needs you also.

Men in this culture are taught how to live—how to get, to have, and to do all the things they're told represent what a man should be. The job. The house. The family. And let's not forget the car! All of these represent the things a man is supposed to have in order to be acknowledged and accepted.

But what does it really mean to be a man? Depending on who's asked, the answer could be anything from a rich and powerful influential leader of people to a gun-toting, foul-mouthed renegade. To a 90 percent certainty, though, most of the definitions would lean toward *having* or *doing* a particular thing. Rarely would someone respond that manhood is a *state of being*. No, being a man is generally defined by what a man *does*. Doing is *physical;* it's *action*. For men, doing is the defining function of the masculine persona. *Being,* on the other hand, is *spiritual*. It's an inward movement, a consciousness of the natural essence. Few men are taught the true spiritual essence of their masculinity.

The men I've known were never taught how to *be* men. They were taught what men *do*. Because we live in a world where we judge people by their actions, being and doing are often confused. So if you don't *do* enough, or *do* it in the right way, you're just not enough as a person. And when you're not enough—when you feel worthless and unvalued, when you feel that nobody sees you for who you are—not only do you get angry and afraid and break out into all sorts of harmful actions, but you lose your fundamental anchor and identity of being a beloved child of the Divine.

My brother was taught to *do*. He was taught to compete. He had to walk tall, run fast, throw far in order to outdo his competitors. My father taught him all he knew about doing. Yet as far as my dad was concerned, my brother could never do enough. My grandmother would say, "Let the boy be!" My father's retort was always, "If you had your way, he'd be a sissy!"

There's that doing and being again: men must *do* whatever is necessary not to *be* a sissy. A sissy, as that label relates to men, is a man who is quiet, meek, noncompetitive, nonaggressive—a man whose masculinity is questionable and up for grabs.

Yet you can describe spirit the same way—a nonphysical essence that represents (in and around all of us) all that God is. Spirit is quiet, noncompetitive, nonaggressive, and invisible. It's also genderless and colorless, making no distinction between male and female, Black and White.

When I think about my brother and his peers, my father and his peers, I see that for them being a man wasn't only what they did; it was also their posture, the manner in which they moved. It was a physical, or outer, demonstration of manliness. I don't recall ever hearing anyone tell my brother that he was good inside. Any support he got was for what he *did*. I don't remember ever hearing about his mission, his purpose, or his everlasting connection to his Creator. What my brother was taught was bravado. Being cool. Walking away.

In light of all these expectations and all this instruction, in light of the fact that men are judged by their *do,* not by their *who,* it's understandable that many of you have developed some very bad habits. Those of us who watch you struggle with what you've been taught (but haven't yet figured out) know that old habits are hard to break. We know how many of you think poorly of yourselves, expect little for or from yourselves. We know that many of you are totally unaware of the spirit within you and of Spirit's purpose in your life. We know that many of you recognize that Spirit contributes to your life, but we also know that you can't figure out what to do with it or about it—especially not since you're also trying to meet all the needs that you feel have been placed on your shoulders.

So those of us watching your struggle either cheer you on or throw our hands up, helplessly disgusted when you don't make it, when you don't get the things you're competing for. We, the onlookers, forget that we're the same ones who aren't listening to (or at least aren't *hearing*) what you're trying to say. We've been looking at your actions, at what you *do,* and we've failed to recognize that you were taught what to *do* rather than how to *be.*

It's my duty as a woman and as a teacher to recognize the fear in men that comes from taking your value from outer things that can fail, fall short, be repossessed. I must acknowledge the anger and look beyond the hostility that comes out of all this to see the truth of who men are.

I also must take responsibility for the fact that who you are reflects a part of who we, the women in your lives, are. Your spirits often reflect the angry, hostile parts of ourselves. When we shift our thoughts and feelings, so too will you. Prayer and forgiveness are responsible ways that we women can assist you, the men we love, in finding your souls. Prayer and forgiveness are necessary steps toward creating the balance, harmony, and peace needed to overcome the challenges of the expectations we put on men in this society.

But first we need to see clearly just what those expectations are. One of the ways in which I can take responsibility for the mess we're in—men and women alike—is to try to shed some light on the path. This book is my attempt to do just that. In it, you'll read some stories you might see yourself in. They're not simple stories with easy endings, but complicated ones that reflect all the different pulls a man feels as he attempts to be a "real" man in this world. You'll see, I hope, that the rage, the guilt, the shame, and the fear men feel all hold the seeds of amazing personal power and freedom, *if you're willing and ready to do the work these powerful emotions lead you to.*

Although these so-called *negative,* or *toxic,* emotions are the most difficult ones for a man to recognize, acknowledge, and understand, they hold all the energy you need to transform your life from one based on *what you do* to one grounded in *who you are.* Difficult though these emotions can be, I encourage you to look for them (and for their repercussions in your life and relationships). Once you've recognized and identified them, tell yourself the truth about what you feel and how your feelings translate into action. Then ask yourself, Why have I been afraid to acknowledge this emotional aspect of myself? The answer will lead to the understanding required to turn a toxic emotion or painful memory into an amazing inner authority and personal power.

What I hope is that you'll see yourself in these pages and be willing to recognize that your feelings of frustration, anger, rage, shame, and guilt are so toxic that they alter your ability to perceive the truth. Being frightened, angry, and unstable is hard for anyone to accept. Our ego defies such things. We've all been taught that fear is an indication of weakness, and men don't easily admit to weakness of any kind. The easiest response to the threat of weakness is to lay blame elsewhere and fight back in defiance. The mind says, *If somebody hits you, hit back.* This is not, however, the way to the real power that lies underneath the anger and fear.

The transformation process is an internal, spiritual one, regardless of your gender. If you want to transform your life, you must be willing to explore the depths of your inner self. Change is an inside job. Your work involves a readiness and willingness to reach within and experience the depths of your emotion, because that understanding holds the key that will unlock your power and freedom.

After you've figured out what's going on inside you, you have to be willing and able to clean the bad stuff out. I offer power tools in this book to do just that. The bad new is, it's often dark "in there." Most of us are afraid of the dark, afraid of what we can't see but can sense around us. The good news is, power is born in darkness.

Some of you will say, "I don't know what to do!" That's where the process of this book comes in. If you're willing to employ the steps shown here, you'll change your life and bring about a deep, rich, and independent existence. Don't be afraid of the dark and of the ugly emotions that lurk there, because they hold the secret of your transformation.

You're endowed with the ability to master yourself. This ability is a function of your connection to your Creator. Spiritual mastery is a process of becoming consciously aware of your thoughts, consciously accountable for your actions, and consciously mindful of the connection between what you feel and how you act. Spiritual mastery requires listening to your inner self, your thoughts and feelings, for guidance. It requires being able to recognize when ego, not Spirit, is motivating your actions. When you acknowledge that you're connected to the divine mind of the Creator, and not to societal expectations that you aren't meeting (and never could), you'll master your ability to hear your spiritual voice. With that mastery, you'll rise up from here.

Mastery in any area of life—whether it's sports or business or Spirit—requires a willingness to stand by certain intangible principles. In the spiritual realm, mastery means standing on faith, trusting in the process of divine order, knowing that in pursuit of truth, by virtue of harmlessness, all situations will evolve to further the well-being of everyone involved. Spiritual mastery means being in control of the demands of the physical self in pursuit of the development of the spiritual self. When that balance is accomplished, a sense of freedom in life is yours.

My father didn't scream at my mother because he wanted to hurt her or because he thought she was deaf. Sometimes he screamed because he believed that he was losing control of her and what she was doing. Other times he screamed because his ego, his physical mind, was offending him.

E-g-o is an acronym for Easing God Out, which is what happens when the physical mind rather than the spiritual mind controls the body. When the ego senses a loss of control, it triggers in your body a need to act. You'll feel in control of your life when you realize that true mastery requires that you clearly see what motivates every action you take. You must recognize and be willing to admit your motivations to yourself in order to make better choices.

This work is best done by looking at others, because when we're feeling bad, we rummage in our bag of tricks for something that will distract us from having to look at ourselves. That's human nature. We blame; we see ourselves as victims. Unless you're both willing and ready to name and claim your emotions, and to recognize what actions and events come out of them, mastery (and the power and freedom that come with it) will remain beyond your grasp.

This book contains portraits of seven men. Look at each one of them. Then get a mirror and look at yourself reflected back. If what you see could use some improvement, use the transformational power tools in this book to name and claim your feelings—the good, the bad, and the ugly. If you're beaten up enough by your life, then you're ready to change. Like the phoenix, you can rise up from your valley, out of the ashes of the crash-and-burn of the past, to claim your true identity and power. This is what I wish for you and for the women in your life who love you.

1

Up from Here

If you're holding this book in your hands, it's a pretty safe bet that there are things in your life that aren't working for you. Maybe it's the job, or the fact that there *is* no job. Maybe it's your relationship with someone in your family—your mother, perhaps, or your child—or maybe it's the woman who is (or isn't) in your life. Maybe it's a feeling of powerlessness or a dislike of what you see in the mirror. I don't know which of these it is, but I *do* know this: this book is here to give you courage, willingness, and tools to address and change those things that are holding you back, keeping you down and grounded, and preventing you from realizing your potential and becoming the divine person you're meant to be!

Right off, I can tell you two things to make these changes easier. First, if and when you see yourself in the pages of this book (and see the things about yourself that you try never to reveal to anybody), you don't have to tell anyone you're looking at yourself. Second, if you can't yet admit that you're seeing yourself in this book, you can recognize someone *else*—a friend, a brother—and learn from him.

This is what I hope for you: that you'll be able to see that where you are now, dark as it may be, has a purpose. It's the beginning place, and all journeys to satisfaction and fullness need someplace to start from. When you're low, there's nowhere to go but up—and together we can go up from here.

This business of coming from a dark place to a light one is a very personal process. It takes place between you and yourself in the privacy of your own mind and the sacredness of your own heart. The only evidence that you've even read this book will be what happens in your life when you put its principles into practice. People are going to look at you and say, "What have you been doing? You're doing *something* different!" This book is about looking at the secret places, the silent places, the wounded places, the crying places within you. If you're now ready to acknowledge them, and accept them and embrace them, then you can heal.

One concept of healing is that it's the application of love to the wounded places, the places where there's darkness or ignorance. All of us in the human race have dark places inside, places that have been injured, chipped, cracked, stretched almost to breaking. These places require infinite amounts of love. When they get that love—when we learn to take the power and strength of our own love and apply it to those places—healing occurs.

It's important to realize that the fact that there's a dark or wounded side of you doesn't mean there's anything *wrong*. It means only that you've been living out your own spiritual curriculum, learning your own lessons, doing your own thing—just as the Divine's plan of your life would have you do. But there comes a day of graduation when you have to move, progress, elevate, or get promoted from one grade to the next, and that movement requires shedding light on the darkness, treating the wound, refinishing the cracks—and that's what healing is.

Love isn't anything that we *do;* rather, it's who we are and what we are. Our lessons, our trials, our experiences are all divinely designed to bring us to that place within ourselves where nothing exists but love.

This book will give you the courage, the strength, the tools, and the process for looking at the dark places inside yourself. The goal of this book is to encourage, assist, and support you in acknowledging that those dark, broken, chipped places exist, and in the process to give you the tools, information, and encouragement you need to bring healing light, balance, and peace to those places.

Reclaiming the Male Spirit

I'm not my brother's keeper; I *am* my brother. And if *I* need healing, my brothers need healing. Everywhere we look today we see that things are changing, people are changing, our approach to life and living is changing. It's not that we have to get rid of what we have and who we've become, but we certainly have to approach our lives differently. The Native Americans talk about walking gently through life, and that's a message we need to hear and heed. We as a human race haven't walked gently through our lives. Not only have we walked harshly on the earth and been harsh with one another, we've brutalized *ourselves*. In doing so, we've allowed (and sometimes even invited) others to join in on the process.

It takes courage to really look at yourself in order to determine what's going on in your life. Only then can you glimpse what's behind your unexamined emotions and recognize the damage they've caused you and others. It's my intention to remind you of what you already have: you have the innate goodness of Spirit within you. I want you to know who you already are: you're one in whom God is well pleased! It's also my intention to show you that much of your goodness has been covered and cloaked and undermined and stepped on. It's my prayer that you'll be able to recognize that you've done a lot of the stepping yourself, because only with that information will you be able to make better choices in the future.

Based on my experience with men, I believe that all too often they view life through a brutal, terrorizing screen. I'm aware that this outlook often comes from the brutality of their personal experiences, the terror of their early family interactions. If we grow up with hurt, then we act or react from that damaged place, with that damaged vision. Being left alone in our heads *without adult supervision,* we come up with things that terrorize us.

Terror on its own would be bad enough, but it generally causes us to limit our beliefs and expectations about who we are and who we might become. Those limiting beliefs about our lives and ourselves (and our limited views of reality) cloud how we look at everything and everyone, not to mention how we see the world. When we're reminded who we are (divine creatures with powerful spirits!), when we're reminded why we're here (to achieve our unique place on this planet), and when we've seen how we got knocked off our course, then we can figure out how to get back on track. This is what I mean by reclaiming the male spirit.

Understanding How Emotions Transform Us

Emotion is the energy that moves us. In fact, the very word *emotion* has *motion* in it! The investment that you put into your emotional being determines *if* you move, *when* you move, and *why* you move.

Sometimes our emotions develop in ways that cause us harm. Other times we unknowingly misuse good and healthy emotions to hurt ourselves. Nobody wakes up one morning and says, "Let me abuse myself, lower my esteem, and abase myself." But we learn by what we see and experience and perceive. Those things then become our programming. Once that programming is in place on our hard-drive, all we have to do is push a button and the function occurs automatically. And our emotions provide the energy that moves those programs!

So many things we do to hurt ourselves, we do without even thinking; they've become habitual. We lie when we're afraid, for example. We attack when we're made to feel wrong. We run when we feel overwhelmed. We hide when we feel inadequate. We wait for external validation when we haven't developed our inner authority. Those who loved us when we were young—those who raised us, guided us, reared us—were doing the best they could. What neither they nor we realized was that *their* hard-drives had kinks in them too. Watching those people and vowing that we wouldn't be like them didn't help us, because few of us were taught how to *be;* we knew only how to *do.*

So now, in order to change our lives for the better, we have to rewrite the programs that were given to us through pain and fear. We need to create and then execute more realistic, more Spirit-centered programs in our minds, lives, and relationships. The keys to writing these new programs are locked up in the emotions that we've never been taught to express.

Walking Gently on the Earth

If your behavior isn't getting you what you want, you have to look at how you go about trying to get things. We often demand, command, and dictate. We speak harshly. We walk away when thwarted. We act tough even when we don't feel that way.

The alternative—walking gently on the earth—has gotten a bad rap among men. But taking a softer approach isn't about being a wimp. It's about having command over yourself and using your emotions for your own good and the good of others. Walking gently in your life means that you know you're so divine and so important that everything you do impacts somebody else, and therefore you want to act with love, compassion, and consciousness so that you don't contribute to the destruction of someone else.

If some portion of your programming, lifestyle, and functioning is detrimental to you because the people who raised you, guided you, and educated you walked harshly instead of gently, then you've been affected by what they did. Likewise, what you do and how you do it affects everyone and everything you come into contact with.

While who you are, what's happened to you, and what you've done can't be undone, it can be transformed. You can't go back and undo; you can only start from where you are. But you *can* learn to live in a better way. You *can* be transformed.

Truth and Transformation

In this book, you're going to read some stories. Some will feel familiar. Some will look like people you know. What these stories are going to show is how we've covered up the essential truths of our lives and our being. We need to get at those essential truths if we hope to make things better. We also need what I call power tools for change—and this book will give you those. It will also give you the secrets of the power of emotion—a power can either hold you back or set you free.

The stories presented here will help you acknowledge your own behavior truthfully, provided you can see your actions (or the actions of others you know) in the people the stories describe. The stories will allow you to believe in who you are and help you forgive yourself and others so that you can get past the hurt and see how essential you are as a human being.

If you're like most of us, you don't believe that who you are is important. And yet you *are* important; in fact, you're divine! And what you do is important. Even if it's something as seemingly small as being a safe driver and not darting in and out in your new Camaro to scare an old lady in her Delta 88. Or holding the door and not letting it slam behind you even though you're late. Or putting up with your pain-in-the-ass mother-in-law so that you can teach your observant son how to be kind.

Transformation has happened when you realize on every single level how absolutely important you are, when you start really *believing* in your importance. You may not have your own company or your own TV show. You may not own the place you sleep in every night. But you matter. What you do matters, and what happens to you matters. Once transformation has happened, you begin to act each and every day from that deep knowledge that you're important.

There are transformation plans in this book that can take you to that place of life-changing knowledge. By using these plans, you'll be able to find what you've lost in the middle of your anger and disappointment and put that crucial sense of importance back to work in your life.

The transformation plans presented here are going to challenge people who are results oriented, because the plans are based on a *process* of change. Too often we want to simply go from point A to point B. Sometimes that works, but more often it doesn't. Often we lie about results, saying that we've gotten to point B when we're still miles away.

Let's say that you've been married three times and now have a fourth wife ten years your junior who does everything you want. Have you really gotten to an ideal place finally, or does it just look like it? Have you learned from the past, or is your rage so terrifying to this present wife that she's submissive in order to keep away from it? Your attentive wife may look good from the outside, but only you and she know the truth. If you have a problem with rage, you're going to have to go into that emotion and use it to transform you and your life. And do it now before that submissive fourth wife packs her bags!

Real change will happen when you can tell the truth quietly to yourself and see that the truth wants only to encourage you, support you, uplift you; it doesn't aim to embarrass you, blame you, or accuse you. There are various tools—the power tools that I mentioned earlier—that work hand in hand with telling the truth. Willingness, awareness, acknowledgment, confession, acceptance, surrender, forgiveness, understanding, commitment, responsibility, right action, and stillness—all these help reveal the truth, and they help truth heal the wounded. These transformational tools are key; they all work together.

Telling the truth—the truth about what you feel, about how you've participated in what's going on in your life, about the role you've played in both your failures and your successes—will free you. Telling the truth isn't blaming or accusing or resorting to self-victimization. Arising from a place of compassion, it's the honest admission of "This is how I thought I should do it, this is why I thought that, and this is what happened as a result. I see now that it could have been done better, but back then this is how I saw it and this is what I did."

Once you acknowledge the truth of the various situations in your life, you can begin to clear away all the alibis that stand in the way of your freedom and true power. You can then learn how to take responsibility for your feelings, examine your choices, and move off your present position—the one that feels so right but that somehow cuts you off from your true power.

The Promise of the Process

Each story in this book will be followed by steps in the process that will make clear how to turn the lostness, the hurt, and the angry emotions into powerful, skillful tools for living. I can promise you that if you keep an open mind, allowing the truth of the stories in, a number of life-changing, life-affirming things will happen to you:

1. *You will begin to feel that you're worth your own attention and time and energy.* It's liberating to feel as worthy of

your own time, your own attention, your own energy as are your mother, your kids, your wife, and your job.

2. *You will sense a deep inner communion of mind and body as things begin to happen inside you.* I can't predict exactly what you'll feel, but I know that you'll get a burst of renewed energy, because it takes enormous effort to cover our hurt rather than heal it. Think of a sixteen-year-old boy who is hurt and trying not to act hurt. Imagine how hard he works just to put on a good front.

3. *When you begin to see and treat yourself differently, everything and everybody around you will shift.* People are going to respond in kind to your changes: they'll start seeing you differently and treating you differently too. As a result, you'll find that the things you used to have to scream about and bang on and demand begin to come to you under grace. Because when you bring yourself into alignment and attunement with the truth of your inner being—which is really the energy that the world was built upon—you don't have to work so hard to get what you want.

4. *Once you're aligned and know who you are and have gotten better by practice, you'll gain a confidence that can't be*

shaken. Michael Jordan knew that he was a basketball player from an early age. He never walked out on the court saying, "I can't play basketball." He knew that if he'd practiced and rested well and supported himself with food or prayer or whatever, when he hit the court he'd be able to play well. Sure, he'd have to work for it, but there was no question about what he could or couldn't do.

Not everybody has that unshakable sense of themselves. You can be a lawyer, for example, with all the necessary credentials, and even after a win in the courtroom still doubt whether or not you're a good lawyer. If your heart isn't in it, passing the bar doesn't mean much. Is your heart in serving your clients, or is it in wearing the fancy suits and making the money—in other words, the *props* of law? Maybe you went to law school, as I did, because you hoped that your degree would give you an image of power (as opposed to power itself). During my years with the law, I was never sure that I was a good lawyer. It didn't matter if I won or lost a case, because I wasn't living from the truth of my being.

5. *The transformation process will give you relief; it will enable you to stand in your authenticity, the truth of your*

being. You'll no longer have to pretend to be someone you're not. And this will be true throughout all the levels of your being. There's the physical level, which is what we see, what materializes; there's the mental level, which is what we think (which supports what materializes); and there's the emotional level, which is what we feel (which feeds our thoughts and is fed by our thoughts, and which, like our thoughts, can show up in our physical world).

These levels are the ones we have control over, but the truth of our being is on yet another level: the spiritual level. When we're aligned and no longer pulled out of shape by the behavior that comes from the powerful emotions of fear, rage, shame, and guilt, relief floods through the mental, physical, and emotional levels.

6. *Finally, you will gain a sense of true power and true freedom to be what and who you're supposed to be.* You will be transformed from someone stuck in old, harsh habits to someone with integrity in his life.

The reason we concentrate on the emotions for transformation is that emotional energy, not thought, is what creates movement in our body. You can *think,* "I'm strong; I'm powerful," but if you *feel* afraid, that fear is going to determine whether and how you move.

I think of a six-foot-two athletic friend of mine who goes to the gym three times a week. This fit and hefty guy hit me on the head with a three-pound book the other day because he was scared of the bee that had lighted on me! This friend is very intelligent, mind you. He should have known that hitting someone on the head wasn't a very smart thing to do under any circumstance. In fact, he probably *did* know that. But it wasn't his mind that was in control; it was his feelings. The emotion of fear, prompted in this case by a bee, blinded him to all reason, and he took the book in both hands and *wham*. There I was on my knees while he was trying to see where the bee had gone! Our emotions blind us in that way all too often.

But emotions are also the energy that *moves* us, as I noted earlier. They—*not* our thoughts—are the keys to our transformation. We can affirm ourselves into oblivion, reciting affirmations until our tongue falls out. And yet if we don't believe, if we can't *feel* in our gut that we can do some particular thing, it isn't going to get done. In other words, we can't sustain any success with our heads alone. Success happens only through our feelings.

This book requires you to take a probing and honest look at your actions and your life. Those outer manifestations are a function of your inner reality. Because rebirth happens from the inside out, if you want to change you have to look at what shows up on the outside and track it back in. This book will show you how to transform your life with the energy of your emotions, allowing you to reclaim your truth, purpose, and place in the universe.

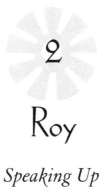

2

Roy

Speaking Up

Let me tell you about a man named Roy. Roy grew up under the influence of a very authoritarian father. His father set the example that if you yell loudly enough about something you want, and if you threaten enough, you'll get what you want. However, there was no room in the family for anyone but Roy's father to make any noise. As a result, Roy had very little voice: he was never able to speak up for himself, to express himself.

As a teenager and young man, Roy felt lost. By the age of nineteen, he was expected to be out in the world on his own, earning a living and taking care of himself. He managed okay, but by his early twenties he was still clueless, drifting from job to job and woman to woman. He would start each new job full of ideas, trying to find his voice, his identity, but because he had no positive role model, his identity never took shape.

Role models are very important for men. Both men and women learn by doing, but men, I think, watch their models a little more closely, because the things that make a man are much more subtle. Women are overt—they cook, they clean, they have babies. But what is it that makes a man a man? Unfortunately, men usually learn that crucial information by what it is they *haven't* done.

Roy couldn't find his voice because the only male voice he was familiar with was a scream. And what do you do when someone screams? There are really only two choices: scream back or clam up. Screaming didn't serve him at work, where the right to scream was always held by someone else, someone higher up the ladder. And with women? Forget it. He went through so many of them that he couldn't remember all of their names. After a first polite date or two, he would demand his way in a raised voice, stamp his foot, and sooner or later every woman walked. His only blueprint for behavior came from his father, who bullied and threatened his mother. Roy's father didn't *listen* to women; he pontificated at them. Other than as a sounding board, the older man had no use for women outside the bedroom.

Now, at twenty-four, Roy has a live-in girlfriend and a baby boy he adores. He works for a national electronics warehouse chain and gets considerable satisfaction from his job. He began there in inventory and has since moved up to managing one area of the floor. The store manager is only a couple of years older than he is and has a great deal of ambition. He also has strong ideas about how things should be done, and he doesn't hesitate to tell Roy what to do and how to do it. Roy doesn't always agree with the manager but isn't sure how to express his disagreement.

Roy likes his job but is worried that he isn't as skilled as some of his co-workers, who seem smooth and confident. They somehow get the high-ticket items to sell, while Roy wastes his time in the lower end. They seem to know how to deal with the controlling manager better than Roy does. But then, the manager has it in for him—or so it seems to Roy.

Instead of looking to others for direction—perhaps one of those co-workers he admires—Roy seeks consolation in a bottle of alcohol. Drinking eases the pain. The pain of fearing that he's not going to do it right and will get yelled at. The pain of fearing that somebody's going to recognize his pain and shame him for it. Or the worst pain of all—not knowing what to do and how to do it, and not having the voice to ask.

When Roy has been drinking, he can speak up just fine. He can tell everybody exactly where he is and how he feels. Alcohol gives him courage. Other men find courage in the act of trying and succeeding at something, but not Roy. Although he won't admit to a dependence on drink, Roy recognizes it deep inside. Every time Roy tries to make a difference at work—tries to make a contribution all his own, in his own way—he has to undo it and do it again the manager's way. And alcohol is his only consolation.

One day there's an accident at work in Roy's area. Thousands of dollars of equipment lie in ruins and two people are sent to the hospital. The manager of the store asks to test Roy's urine, to see whether his judgment might have been impaired at the time of the incident. Roy refuses because he knows that he's been drinking beer and smoking weed.

The choices, as Roy sees them, are these: either let his employer test him—which, in his mind, means he'll get caught out and lose his job—or become arrogant and angry and walk away. Roy chooses arrogant and angry (even though the human resources manager offers to get him into rehab rather than push for dismissal if the test should reveal impairment), and he walks away.

But he doesn't go quietly. He's angry as all get-out that anyone would question him, and he's more angry still at the thought that someone might find out not only that he was smoking pot but also that he is just plain inferior to the others, who aren't being tested. So before he walks he tells all his co-workers exactly what he thinks of each and every one of them.

When Roy gets home he realizes that any hope he might have had for the future with that company is dead. Maybe, he thinks, he should have swallowed his pride and dealt with it head-on. But as quickly as that thought comes, he dismisses it. Hey, didn't he know better than that manager? Wasn't it the manager's fault that his area was set up in a way that allowed an accident to happen? Hadn't he himself wanted to do things differently? Assholes! Who needs them?

Talking to the Man in the Mirror

When you can't say what you need to say, what's in your heart, no one can see who you are or give you what you need. That's the problem Roy faces. Having grown up with every thought and movement controlled by his father, he now sees only two ways of dealing with people he perceives as having power over him: he either fights (which he knows won't work, because it never, ever worked with his dad) or self-destructs, imploding in silence and deadening his pain with alcohol and smoke. Because Roy can't face the manager, he walks away. Because Roy has no coping mechanism for dealing with anyone in charge, he avoids such dealings.

When Roy is questioned by an authority figure, the experience triggers all the rage that's been pent up inside him since his childhood. And it doesn't take direct questioning either: whenever he feels his personal space or personal power threatened in any way, the anger comes forward. But since he tries not to be outwardly aggressive, his anger shows up in arrogance. Roy feels that he shouldn't have to answer to others, so he doesn't. In his mind, it's just that simple.

Roy's response to questioning, though self-destructive, has some very real survival roots. When he didn't walk away as a boy, he was assaulted verbally or even physically by his father. He learned that lesson well, developing an attitude of arrogance to save some shred of personal dignity. Now, though, with his father no longer a danger, Roy's "No one is going to get in my face" attitude has backfired. He's lost not only his job but all his prospects for the future.

Worse yet, he loses his girlfriend and his son when he gets home. Reading disaster on his face, his girlfriend asks him what happened and whether he's high. "High?" he yells, outraged. Whose side is she on?—the ungrateful bitch. Hasn't he told her that the manager had his head up his ass? And now she's questioning him?

Well, one more look at the glassy eyes and she knows all she needs to know. This is the third time he's come home jobless and loaded and screaming in the short time she's known him. Enough is enough. She doesn't want to stay around for the verbal abuse that she knows will follow, so she heads for the bedroom to pack.

But Roy feels like the victim here. He can't listen to what his girlfriend says because all he hears is her screaming. When she says she's leaving, he tells her to get the hell out, though he feels a knife go through him as he says it. But one look at that bitch's angry face spurs him on. Who needs her? Get out!

Roy's arrogance costs him big this time. He watches from the kitchen table, a smoke in his shaking hand, as the only person he truly loves—his son—is packed up and bundled into his girl-friend's sister's car. He can't even bring himself to go to the door to kiss the boy, because he's using arrogance to mask his fear.

What a mess. He couldn't deal with the manager's questioning so he left in a huff, and now it turns out that leaving wasn't such a hot idea either! It hurts like hell to be off the job and see his family leave.

There are deeper side effects as well. Though Roy probably doesn't think in these terms, leaving causes him to question and doubt himself, his abilities, and his very right to exist. He feels now as he used to feel as a kid after a dressing-down for something he did or didn't do: there's something wrong with who he is.

The approach to life that he learned in childhood cost Roy his sense of self, his sense of personal power, and his sense of personal dignity. All this makes him very angry from time to time, and now that anger has cost him all the things he most wants in life.

Right about now, Roy is feeling pretty out of control. His emotions are calling the shots in his life, and if he wants any mastery, he's going to have to figure out what's going on inside. That's hard to do while in the grip of powerful emotions, but emotions do what they can to help.

All emotions have behaviors that are like symptoms, and Roy is breaking out in a whole bunch of those. If he can see them in himself, they'll lead him to where he needs to go to transform the negative into the positive. He'll then see that anger isn't inherently bad. Indeed, in many circumstances it's appropriate. Furthermore, it contains the power to move him, emotionally.

There are a number of key symptoms of anger. People in the grip of anger do (or feel) the following:

Demand to have their own way

Try to control everyone and everything around them

Have little tolerance for other ideas, other input, other points of view

React in ways that are stronger than the situation demands, because the threat feels out of proportion to the situation—a matter of survival, not just an incident at hand

Feel an energetic in the body that rises up from the gut

Roy certainly would have recognized these behaviors in his father, but his future depends on whether he can see them in himself. He needs to see that, as an adult, he's reacting to the world in the same way he did as a child—and he's brimming with anger as a result.

When Roy was a child, he wouldn't challenge his father or other caregivers. He wouldn't speak his mind or say things in his own defense. But now he's creating in his own life the very things he suffered with as a child. If he's not silencing others, as his father did, he's silencing himself! Unless he's got some very special friends, there's probably no one in his adult life willing to challenge him—willing to say, "You're striking out," when he comes on too aggressive, or "You're wimping out," when he holds his tongue unreasonably.

But even without that feedback, he knows. That's why he's got to tell the truth now. He knows when he's bullying those around him. He knows when he's silencing people who disagree with him. He knows when he's lashing out. He knows when he's walking away. Oh yes, he knows.

Roy needs to see clearly what's going on and take ownership of his feelings and actions if he's to have any hope of turning his life around. He needs to see that what looks like self-righteous anger and arrogance is really fear. He's got to tell the truth about what he feels and find a way to express his feelings honestly and constructively.

Roy is afraid, and he's angry. But what should he do with those feelings? Some fear is appropriate, of course—for all people—as is some anger. When Roy first felt both those emotions, they were appropriate to him too: he was *angry* at his abusive father, and he was *afraid* to express that anger because he could get hurt. But because Roy hasn't gotten past that point, his emotions are no longer appropriate. He has to see that the root of his anger at his boss is his anger at his dad.

That anger has been festering for two decades. But how does he—how does *anyone*—acknowledge, much less express, anger at a father? This is the person who fed and clothed him when he was a youngster. Who's supposed to love him. The person on whom he used to be dependent for his very survival. The person who even now models manhood and right behavior for him. How does he stand in opposition to all that?

Not only is Roy angry, but his inner authority, his inner guidance, and his very masculinity have been undermined. Roy's *who* has become all wired up with his *do;* and now, because he feels undermined by others, he undermines himself even further. He has to find a way to separate his emotional self-image from his actions.

Roy's anger can either stop him or empower him. If the anger is so hot that he isn't willing to touch it, it will seal him in and may, given his makeup, make him depressed. But if he's willing to handle it despite the heat, it holds the seeds of his transformation.

When Roy talks to himself in the mirror, how does he go from the guy who just turned on his heels and kissed his future good-bye, the guy who's still drinking and smoking weed, to someone capable of getting in touch with the power of transformation? Especially right now, when what he really feels is *powerless*. Because when he feels powerless, he gets even more angry.

The answer is simple, though not easy: Roy achieves his transformation through a healing process that can be applied to every man and every woman and every situation in this book (and in this world). That process is based on the power principles, or power tools. These tools are the foundation for all personal transformation.

A Spiritual Toolbox: Using Power Tools

Men are taught that it's not "manly" to be afraid or to demonstrate weakness or emotion. Yet certain emotions, if not expressed, can weaken your physical being. Vulnerability, fear, guilt, shame, resentment, anger—when not acknowledged, these can lessen your ability to perceive circumstances around you, make conscious choices, and respond.

If you're like most men, when certain emotions erupt within your being, you deny them as you were taught. In fact, you deny them even to yourself. It's not just that you don't express them; you don't even acknowledge that you feel them. If you have a tough day at work—maybe a putdown at the hands of a colleague, a complaint about your service from a customer, and a warning about productivity from your boss—you don't recognize and deal with your emotions; you go home and chew out your wife and kids and rant for a while about all the jerks there are in the world. In short, you follow your masculine nature and strike out, blaming others for what they "made" you do, looking to them as the cause of your response or experience. Because the inherent nature of men is to direct activity and energy outward, because masculine energy is an aggressive energy inclined to reach beyond itself, men find looking *within* to be a foreign concept.

And yet only when you're willing to admit that your feelings exist and that you have a right to experience them will you be empowered to choose what to do. Emotions result from experiences. Experiences are temporary: they cannot and do not change who and what you are at the core of your being. Same goes for emotions. So you need to feel them, own them, act in response to them, and then move on.

Will Roy be capable of doing that? Only time will tell. His outward-reaching masculine aggression is working overtime these days, hurting those around him and turning in on himself. There's a place for that aggression, though, a use for that outward energy, but not until Roy can grasp and use the power tools of willingness, awareness, acknowledgment, acceptance, confession, surrender, forgiveness, understanding, commitment, responsibility, right action, and stillness.

Willingness

No amount of information about self-improvement can help you until you're ready to receive that info and apply it to your daily living. I refer to this readiness to accept information and embrace practices leading to spiritual and personal transformation as *willingness*.

When I told a friend of mine that I was writing a book to give men insight into the process of the spiritual transformation of emotions into power, he said, "Good! You're preparing lunch!" I laughed at that apparent non sequitur and asked him what he meant. He explained that providing such a process, and the principles by which to employ it, is like making lunch for a man going off to work. He cautioned me, however, that unless the man is willing to go to work, there's no need to prepare his lunch.

My friend's warning is a good one. Transformation of the mind to a spiritual consciousness takes a great deal of work. It's work the individual must be willing to perform; no one can do it for him. Men must be willing to examine themselves, tell the truth about what they see, make a conscious decision to change, and be committed to take those actions that will facilitate the change.

Some will say, "But I don't know what to do!" That's where the process presented in this book comes in. All that's required of you at the outset is a willingness to employ the steps of the process in every aspect of your life. Ability will follow as surely as day follows night.

Willingness has three primary components:

A recognition of the need for change

A desire to initiate change

Sufficient discipline to maintain change

Recognition of the need for change. If you're going to start the transformation process, you must first recognize the need for change. This doesn't necessarily mean that there's anything much wrong with the way you are. It means simply that you're willing to do better and be better at whatever it is you do.

Desire to initiate change. Willingness also encompasses desire. You may know that you can do better but lack the desire to do so. Perhaps you've made yourself comfortable where you are. Perhaps you've convinced yourself that this is as good as it gets. In that case, the change process won't ever get off the ground. If, on the other hand, the desire is present, you're ready to make a life-changing decision. Is it your conscious desire to undertake a course of action that will ultimately result in mental, emotional, and spiritual evolution? Do you feel compelled to make your spiritual health, emotional well-being, and physical advancement a priority in your life—not sometime in the vague future, but *now?*

Sufficient discipline to maintain change. If you decide to initiate personal change, you'll need tremendous discipline. I know *I* did. In fact, one of the major challenges I faced on my own spiritual journey was discipline. Remaining convinced that I should do certain things in a particular way, consistently, even when I couldn't see the results immediately, was a challenge. Whether it was prayer, meditation, reading, or training my mind to think a new way and my mouth to speak a new way, finding the discipline to continue was quite difficult.

I was willing, yes, but I was also undisciplined. It was so much easier to struggle along, living on the edge, putting out fires as they presented themselves, than to spend fifteen minutes a day in quiet contemplation. It wasn't until my desire for change and my decision to work toward change were laced with discipline that I became consciously willing to do what was necessary.

When I became not only willing to start but also disciplined enough to stick to my decision, I reaped benefits from daily practice with all the power tools described here. I saw evidence of the principles underlying those tools manifesting as tangible conditions in my life. In the end, the ability to produce in life that which you want is a reflection of the degree of discipline you exert. For that reason, you need to be willing to *practice* using the power tools. You must believe that they'll work for you. You must employ them with all your energy and all your soul.

Let's take another look at Roy and see where he stands in regard to the power tool of willingness. This isn't a tool he yet has in his arsenal, that's for sure. And he can't learn to wield it until he allows his anger to come forward into the light, allows himself to really *feel* it. That means overcoming the fear of what his anger can do. He has to see that anger is a double-edged sword, capable of good as well as evil.

Roy has been told all his life that anger is wrong. You can't be mad at Daddy. You can't be mad at Mommy. You can't be mad at these people who supported you but have spent half their time angry at you! Don't do it: Don't talk back. Don't look at me. Don't challenge me. Don't question me.

It's tough to be ready and willing when Roy is afraid of the anger. He's afraid of what he will do if the anger comes out, even though it bursts from him every now and then whether he's screaming or yelling or slapping somebody or insisting. . . or, when it comes out in the flip side of anger, depression. Roy gets angry because he has no voice and that makes him feel powerless. That's what really happened to Roy. Whenever a man feels powerless, he's going to get angry.

At first all these admonitions were external—spoken by parents, teachers, whoever. Gradually, though, Roy internalized them. Now they're inside him. Ironically, the very thing that's causing Roy pain and discomfort—his anger—is the one thing that he was taught he couldn't, *shouldn't,* challenge or question. As a result, his anger is now hurting himself most of all. He needs to find an appropriate way to express his anger, whether it's through exercise, sports, or therapy.

So for Roy, willingness means reaching a place where he's able to sit, drop his hands to the side, and let the anger come up full force. It means allowing himself to relive some of the painful experiences of his childhood. It means being willing to say to the people who were involved in the creation of the anger (whether childhood anger or the recent anger of being questioned on the job) exactly what it is that he feels.

Awareness

Much of what we feel on any particular day has very little to do with what happens to us that day; it's intricately (but subconsciously) connected to what happened in our past. That's why someone can say something apparently innocuous to us, and we hit the roof over it.

When people push our hot-buttons, they trigger feelings and memories that lie below our level of awareness. We respond to people, events, and situations as if we were still living in the past. We flare up because of things we experienced yesterday or yesteryear. Our boss reminds us of someone who treated us badly, so we snap at him. Our insurance agent talks to us the way our ex-wife did, so we hang up on her.

Because of that subconscious link with the past, when we respond to someone in anger we're often totally unaware of our reasons. We think we're hot under the collar about the other person, but it's not him or her really; it's us responding to old stuff of which we're completely unaware. All the other person did was touch a sore spot, open an old wound, push a button we weren't aware existed.

That's exactly what happened with Roy. Every time he talked to a person in authority, he heard his father's voice preaching at him. Every time he talked to a woman, he heard his father's voice responding in his own.

So what Roy needs now is *awareness*. If he's willing and ready to feel his feelings, he's already heading in the right direction. His feelings will lead him to awareness, if he listens well.

Most of us need pain to become aware. A growing boy isn't aware that his shoes are too small until he feels the pinch on his toes, for example. Spiritual pain is a messenger too. Have you ever told yourself that your life isn't the way you want it to be? Have you ever asked yourself, What's wrong with me? What's wrong with what I'm doing? Something in your experience brought you here. Something that didn't go your way. And that something will lead you to awareness.

Through failure and loss, Spirit gets your attention and wakes you up. It then makes you aware that it isn't the job or the car or the girl or the money that will transform your sorry state, but Spirit itself. You must be aware of Spirit as it lives within you. You must be aware of the truth that Spirit holds and the truth that surrounds you. You must be aware of the role that the spiritual principles play in your life.

The truth is, no degree of racism, capitalism, oppression, or disparity can alter the inherent power of godliness locked in your spirit. When Roy lost his job, he didn't lose his inner spirit. But he *believed* that he did because he believed the lie that the job was his spirit, that the woman was his spirit, that his masculinity was his spirit. Throughout life, these outer experiences and conditions can alter your state of being by affecting what you believe.

If you believe the lie that these outer things tell you—that they're powerful or will make you powerful—then the lie will inform your life. It will alter it, and that alteration will affect your actions. The physical part of your life, your experiences, will be communicated to your brain through the lie. If the brain is left without the spiritual truth of your real nature to fill it up, then the brain will translate all experiences through the lie.

If the brain is to utilize spiritual qualities rather than filtering everything through the lie, the brain must be spiritualized. In other words, it must be filled with information of a spiritual nature. That's a hard task for men. Because the thought process dominates men, you males tend to think in concrete terms. And yet the spiritual impetus of physical experiences can't be seen, because Spirit isn't tangible. As a result, you men often become locked into the physical perception of your experiences and remain unaware of their (and your) spiritual purpose or significance.

In order to change your mind and shift into the awareness of Spirit, you must be willing to seek and embrace the truth about yourself. You must be willing to examine every experience from an internal frame of reference. In the midst of an experience, you must ask yourself, What am I feeling right now? When have I felt this way before? Under what circumstances? Who was involved? In asking such questions, you become aware of your own internal mechanisms—what turns you on and off.

With every emotion, including anger, the key to mastery and power lies in telling the truth about how you feel and about what happened. Roy may look all grown up, but inside there's still that same little boy who experienced being shut down by his father. The anger that came out of that early experience needs to be validated.

The boss isn't going to do that; he just watched Roy give up a great job and leave him in the lurch. His girlfriend isn't going to do that; she's out of there, kid in tow. That means Roy has to do it for himself. Roy has to look at himself in the mirror and honestly see a few things, each one of which can be used to give himself a sense of true power—power anchored to something bigger than a job, a girlfriend, even a son or a father.

Acknowledgment

Roy needs not only to become aware of his feelings, especially his anger; he needs to put a *name* to what he's feeling as well. He needs to identify the energy inside that says, "I can't say what I want to say; I can't challenge this authority." The anger that he's been suppressing with alcohol and weed needs to step forward and be acknowledged.

Acknowledgment is a key step toward healing. Awareness of your feelings is essential, but it's not enough. You can be fully *aware* of something and fail to *acknowledge* it. Alcohol and substance abusers like Roy are prime examples. They may know that they can't get through the day without a drink or a snort, yet they fail to acknowledge that they're addicted.

Acknowledgment means being in a state of recognition of what you're thinking and feeling. It's the way in which you honor and support your right to be and to feel—a right that society, with its emphasis on the denial of men's inner self, does all it can to repress. Acknowledgment is recognition of the truth. That truth may be painful or frightening; however, it's the path to your emotional freedom and spiritual evolution.

Because acknowledging what you feel goes against all your training, it requires an act of will. However, once accomplished, it's a powerful step. After all, it's almost impossible for any human being to *always* do or say the appropriate thing at the appropriate time. There will always be times, regardless of how rare, that you'll act up or act out in a most inappropriate manner. When you do, acknowledge it. Honor yourself. See it for what it was: a temporary experience—nothing to be ashamed of or feel guilty about.

If you fail (or refuse) to acknowledge inappropriate behaviors, they become anchors around your neck, weighing you down and holding you back. You find yourself getting angry with other people, blaming them for what you did. The ego always finds a way, *some* way, to rationalize inappropriate behaviors that you haven't acknowledged.

When you fail to acknowledge your own shortcomings, you set yourself up to be a victim. You give away your power. On the other hand, when you acknowledge what you've done, how you've responded, you become aware of what it is that's unproductive or harmful about your behavior and have the power to act on that awareness. Knowing that a particular way of thinking or acting out your emotional experience isn't reaping the results you desire, you're empowered to choose differently next time. With that knowledge and empowerment, you open yourself up to be healed.

Acceptance

At the core of every human being is an intangible and indestructible power or force that sustains life. That power is the spark of divinity called Spirit. All human beings are made in the image and likeness of God.

This would be a surprise to Roy just about now, because he's feeling anything but godly. But it's true, and it means that he has the same ability and opportunity everyone else does to change on the spot and bring forth this spiritual nature. Peace, strength, freedom, understanding, total well-being, joy, and love—these are the potentials of God inherent in every human being. These attributes are our birthright. The challenge Roy faces, the challenge we *all* face, is accepting that we possess these attributes and recognizing that they're always actively available to us, ready to be incorporated into our lives.

Unfortunately, Roy, like so many of us, has been socially conditioned to look for and expect the benefits of peace and strength and dignity and power to come from other people, places, and things out in the world, rather than from Spirit. But the fact that he *is* that way doesn't mean that he has to *stay* that way. All of us can learn to draw from Spirit.

We do that through *acceptance,* which involves embracing the truth of Spirit and of spiritual principles. When you embrace the truth, you're released from psychological and emotional turmoil. Whether the truth is of a personal nature or is related to spiritual principles, accepting it eliminates the need to fix the world to suit your needs. Acceptance of a tight and difficult situation as it is on another dimension—a spiritual dimension—makes that tight situation much, much roomier. In that added space, it's easier to make some positive and transforming moves.

Acceptance brings with it an inner knowing that all is well, all is in divine order, even when there's no evidence of order in your immediate world. Acceptance also brings the ability to transcend judgment of right and wrong and of the toxic emotions of fear, anger, shame, and guilt, all of which Roy is feeling right about now. If Roy can master acceptance, if he can see that there's more than the immediate situation at hand, he'll feel immediate relief. Even better, acceptance will free up the power in his emotions so that they can help him become truly powerful and free.

Confession

It's frightening to admit to yourself that you've made a mistake, a poor choice, a bad decision, or that you've behaved irresponsibly. It's even worse to acknowledge such things publicly. When you do confess—even if it's to a close friend or much-loved family member—you open yourself to attack, criticism, condemnation, or abandonment. It's downright humiliating to admit to someone you respect that you're helpless or clueless. Yet it's only through a humble spirit that the light of the Divine can enter. Telling the truth not just to yourself but also to another person opens the doors of your mind to spiritual light and moral strength.

Of course, you have to trust that you won't get hammered the minute you spill the beans. If you suspect that you're still reacting to old information when you deal with people, you'd better go back to the tool of awareness and make sure that you're dealing in real time before you tackle *confession*.

But don't put it off too long. This is really an amazing power tool, confession. It frees the mind of guilt, which in turn shuts down the defense mechanism. When you have no guilt, your self-esteem rises. When you have no need to defend yourself, you have little cause to be angry.

Confession also disarms the adversary. If Roy had gone

home and admitted right off that he'd screwed up, his girl-friend probably would have rallied to his side instead of call-ing the moving company. When you point out your own weaknesses, shortcomings, and human frailties, they can't be used against you. People can't hit you over the head with your own bat unless you let them.

That doesn't mean people will be happy to hear what you have to say. That's okay, because chances are you're not proud of what you've done either. But most likely your worst failing is that you acted in fear and confusion or without enough information. Perhaps you felt desperate or alone and simply panicked. That's what Roy did. That isn't *wrong;* that's *human*.

But the truth still needs to come out. When you confess what you've done, and what you were experiencing at the time you acted, don't let the ego get in there and start to whis-per lies and alibis. After all, in your failure you join the human condition. One of our greatest fears is that if we own up to something we'll be isolated and punished, and yet spiritual law reverses that: when we own up, we're one of many—humanity—and we're rewarded with peace of mind.

And that reward is yours even if the person you confess to chooses not to understand. That's a risk you have to take. And it's worth taking, because even if your mother or your wife puts you out or your best friend stops speaking to you, you'll be in better alignment with the universe than ever before, and only good things can come from that. It's the spiritual law. That's why using confession as a power tool works!

Surrender

Here's a popular concept. (Right!) Mention *surrender* to most people, and what they think of is loss of power, defeat, humiliation. You may think that way yourself. You may think of surrender as *My girlfriend or wife or mother was right and I was wrong.* And it all goes downhill from there. Right? No way. Surrender is one of the most powerful tools in your kit. It sets you free. It puts your faith into action, allies you with Spirit, and, most important, shifts the focus from *doing* to *being.*

If you're tired of being judged by what you do or don't do, what you have or don't have, and want to be seen and judged for who you are as a man, you have to get with this surrender, because it's the short, sure highway to what you desire.

Surrender happens when you stand in the middle of all the crap in your life and can manage to be okay with it. The crap is there, smelling very bad, but you don't give in to fear, resentment, or humiliation. At the most basic level, surrender is an admission that you haven't got a clue what to do or what's coming. It means that you're willing to stop pretending that you don't know what you want. *Sure* you do, and you want it bad. Now stop fighting, and what you want will happen. Roy couldn't do that—he couldn't surrender to the situation and admit that he'd had a part in it all—and as a result, he lost everything.

Surrender is essential to a strong relationship. Without it, both parties are forced to play a cat-and-mouse game. You love her, she loves you, and yet you're both afraid to admit it. After all, that would mean surrender! Because you fear looking weak or being humiliated, you resist the attraction; you fight against what you feel and against each other.

Surrendering to your emotions in a relationship means taking a risk, no doubt about it, but once you surrender—once you enter that emotionally unfamiliar territory—you remove the resistance within you. When the resistance goes, so does a great deal of pain. You come into alignment with Spirit, and you provide Spirit with the energy needed to work on your behalf.

Because so many men believe that they've had few personal victories in their lives, surrendering is a major challenge. This, coupled with the images that surrender conjures up in the mind, makes surrender a very unattractive option. But you know how deceptive appearances can be! Try thinking of surrender this way: surrender is an act of courage and power that creates a shift in the consciousness—from being a disempowered human being struggling to make a way, to being a child of God entitled to the best.

Surrender of the *ego* is what we're talking about. Give it up, man! You get all the power of the universe in return!

Forgiveness

Among the power tools, there are few more versatile and powerful than *forgiveness*—forgiveness of self and of others, of past events and present situations. Forgiveness means giving up the old for the new.

As we saw earlier, old experiences and memories often drive our train without our permission (or even our awareness). Things that stew in us—memories that bring anger, resentment, shame, or guilt—cloud our minds and our judgment of right and wrong, good and bad. These old thoughts take us away from the truth and get us into every manner of trouble. Though invisible, they're more powerful than we are.

The only way to be free of these forces is forgiveness. When we forgive ourselves or someone else, that forgiveness liberates us. The great spiritual pain reliever, forgiveness takes acceptance and pushes it one step further.

Most of us believe that when we forgive others, we're excusing their behavior. We think that to forgive is to admit that what's happened is all right. Quite the contrary. Forgiveness moves you out of the way and opens the way for divine justice to prevail. It takes the responsibility from your shoulders, particularly when the focus of your anger is no longer around. When you forgive, you clear your mental and emotional airwaves so that you can get on with your life.

I urge you to lighten your load. Take all that energy you've been spending on blaming yourself or others, in feeling guilty or pissed, and throw it away. Use the energy instead for your highest good.

Understanding

Understanding isn't really an action; it's a reward. An emotional and spiritual awareness that comes after forgiveness, it creates a shift of energy in your mind, body, and spirit. Understanding signals the conscious acceptance of where you end and Spirit begins; it signals acknowledgment of and willing surrender to Spirit. Understanding is revelation of truth. It's the ability to see beyond the immediate to what's real.

The road to understanding has one major pothole: you must be willing to tell the truth to yourself about yourself. You must be able to accept what you do before you can gain an understanding of why you do it. Clarity is a telltale sign that understanding is right around the corner.

Once you see the truth, accept it. Acceptance of the truth is the path to healing. Understanding is the reward of your willingness to heal.

Commitment

When you know what you want and are willing to admit it to yourself and to the world, even at the risk of being called a fool, you have *commitment*. It's a simple tool, but from it comes both the earlier-described discipline and the soon-to-be-described right action. You can't have either without a soul-deep decision to take all that energy freed up by the other power tools and use it to achieve your desires.

Responsibility

Responsibility is synonymous with power. Taking responsibility is the only way to have power psychologically, emotionally, and spiritually. When you take total responsibility for everything that's going on in your life, you have the power to change those things that you don't like. When you take charge, you make your life different in response to what *you* decide *you* want. In other words, you make conscious, deliberate choices. You're no longer a victim. You now have the power to say no to conditions that don't suit you. It comes down to this: taking responsibility is a reflection of your willingness to do something about what's going on (or not going on) in your life.

If Roy doesn't become ready to take responsibility for his anger, he's going to keep recreating situations where he's the voiceless little boy. He's going to do that at work, and he's going to do that in his personal life. He's also going to attract other people who need to find their voices. He's gotten away with things up until now because he has attracted (and been attracted to) people who've been unwilling to challenge him. What he needs is a friend who's brave enough to let him know when his behavior is inappropriate. Someone's got to support that part of Roy that already knows his behavior doesn't work, is hurtful to self and others.

Whenever you find yourself in a difficult situation, ask yourself, "What did I do to get where I am now? How did I contribute to this situation? What was I thinking? What was

I feeling when I entered this experience?" We all have patterns of thought, emotion, and behavior that are locked into our subconscious mind. These patterns attract experiences that reflect what we believe within and about ourselves. As we saw in our discussion of awareness, you must be willing to examine what you do and why you do it. Then you must also take responsibility for your part of what you see—but without guilt, shame, or blame. When you do so, you enable yourself to make conscious, enlightened, productive choices.

We need to take some responsibility for those who interact with us as well. We saw that people in Roy's life have to remind him when his behavior is inappropriate, especially since he tends to attract people who likewise need to find their voice (whether it's as his oppressor or as his enabler). If you have a Roy in your life, you too have to take some responsibility, because not calling him on his behavior enables him to keep going the way he has been.

Think of it this way. There are two dogs—one snarling, one nice. If you keep feeding the snarling dog, hoping to calm him, tame him, mollify him, what happens? The snarling dog gets stronger and the gentle, nice one starts to waste away. You're not in Roy's life by accident: you sought him out just as he sought you out. Now you can help yourself by helping him. If you call Roy on his behavior, pointing out his responsibility, you'll not only help him see that running will never do anything but drain him and those around him; you'll also save yourself from being pushed around by the irresponsibility of others.

What would taking responsibility entail for Roy? First, the awareness that he's a runner, a hider, that he uses his anger to disguise his feeling of shame over the fact that he isn't man enough (as he sees it) to talk back to his father or anyone in authority. Second, the vigilance to monitor his internal responses so that he can recognize his anger and shame whenever they flare up and can discern what the triggers are. Third, the willingness to believe that responding to his triggers is a matter of *choice*. That's what readiness to change requires.

That's what it requires of all of us. Only if we recognize that our behaviors are the result of free choice can we respond to our varying triggers more constructively. Only then can we make better choices, opting for effective strategies over such behaviors as walking away, striking out, or becoming silent and depressed.

Right Action

Right action is the power tool that makes it all happen. It converts all the emotions into the power and freedom men seek. It makes flesh into Spirit. It's alchemy!

Right action, as the label implies, means doing the right thing. If you're angry and resentful, as Roy was, you attempt to control people and situations. No one can take right action in that frame of mind! But if you've used the preceding power tools effectively, you've gotten yourself to the place where you can see a choice in what you do and can choose what's best for you and others; you can choose the right action. And when you *do* right, you get the reward of *feeling* right. You're free!

Don't get me wrong. Right action doesn't mean that you won't stumble sometimes, maybe even fall flat on your face. It doesn't mean that you'll become rich and famous. It means that, whatever happens, you'll accept the experience as a challenge and encouragement to grow, not as an excuse to give up or to beat up on yourself or someone else.

If your intentions are clear and good, right action will eventually manifest the result you desire!

Stillness

Stillness is the art of not doing. It's the practice of faith and trust and belief turned into tangible experience. It has to do with making decisions and not judging yourself afterward as right or wrong, good or bad. Stillness comes when you can be who you are, right where you are, and know that there's a way out of no way. When you have "no where" to turn, stillness is the realization that your help is "now here," in the form of Spirit.

Stillness allows you to see that with the help of Spirit and your power tools, you can regain all the power you've been giving away for years. It gives you the freedom to live in the moment, liberated from all the angers and resentments of the past, free of all the alibis and excuses and blaming.

Knowledge Equals the Freedom to Choose

All of the power tools are essential if you want to use the power of your emotions to transform your life, though not all tools are needed in all situations. All of them in combination give you knowledge. But only if you *use* them. Your success as a human *being,* rather than a human *doing,* rests on your ability to grasp and use these tools. Until you believe that you have the power to make choices, you can't respond with consciousness and deliberation to the choices you do make. Until you assume responsibility for your choices and actions, you can't experience a sense of personal power. Most important, until you integrate your *actions* with the truth of who you are, you can't experience change. That's what all the power tools work up to: action that creates real change. A man can think he wants to change, swear he wants to change, even plan on changing, but until he *acts* in new ways, nothing constructive happens.

Let's look at Roy again. He can go through everything we've talked about here—recognition of his anger, awareness of how it controls him, and so on—but until he takes all that knowledge about himself and how he reacts and makes different, better, choices, the energy of all his negative emotions will pull him back down deep into the pit he's struggling to climb out of. Only if Roy uses his new knowledge to shape new action can he regain the power that resides in his anger and shame. He must choose to use the power of his emotions rather than allow it to use him.

Roy has to start by choosing to express his anger straight on rather than channeling it off into some indirect form of expression. If he can't immediately speak honestly with the important people in his life, he can gain practice and confidence through journaling or therapy. He's got to find a way to get what's in there out, and to express his feelings honestly.

He has to be willing to say to the people in his life that he's angry, that he's hurt, that he feels as if no one sees him for who he is; and then he has to say who that is. By acknowledging not just to himself but to others where he is, he can take all the energy that's been hiding in the anger and turn it outward to change the outer circumstances that reinforce his feelings of powerlessness. Using the anger to find his voice in an appropriate way will change his world. It will stop him from attracting situations and people that make him feel muted, invisible, powerless. If he acknowledges his feelings in a journal, to a friend, to a loved one, or to a boss, then he can choose how he wants to act instead of having the shame and fury choose for him. And once he finds a small voice within, it will get louder as he reaches out to others—other men, the women closest to him, perhaps a psychotherapeutic professional.

As his voice grows in volume and stature, he'll learn to routinely take right action. When he feels a surge of shame or anger, he'll learn to take a deep breath, drop his hands to the side, and keep his mouth shut until he's cooled off. He may have to talk to that angry little boy within, acknowledge him, saying, "I know you're in there. I feel your anger. Now I'm going to take you by the hand and we're going to go this way." In every adult male who's experiencing anger outwardly, there's a six-year-old having a temper tantrum inside. The adult has to step over the six-year-old and say, "Okay, I'm leaving!"

So that anger he finds can lead Roy to a place he could never get to before. It can help him to find his voice and express himself. To ask for what he wants. To think about how he feels, knowing that it doesn't have to go that way. The thing about anger is that the voice was never expressed, or when it was, it didn't go the way he thought it should go. Somebody was saying who you are or what you wanted or what you did was wrong. So being able to move through the anger will get you to know that you can have this feeling, you can have this difference, and it doesn't have to go your way, and it doesn't mean that you are less than a person or less than a man.

We can all learn from Roy. His primary lesson is that the inner response is absolutely key. Don't say you're not angry when you are. Don't say you feel good when you don't. Don't deny *any* feeling, good or bad. But don't let a feeling rule you either. Don't let the six-year-old's temper tantrum determine the adult's action.

The transformative power of anger and other strong emotions means that you ultimately get the power you were looking for in the first place—power not just over the situation but over yourself. Untamed anger is all about the violent and aggressive control of others. What you want to do is turn that control toward yourself.

There are three C's that can help you regain your life: control, cooperation, and compromise. If you *control* your responses, *cooperate* with those around you, and *compromise* as needed, you'll ultimately hold your own reins. That's really what it's all about; it's not about anybody else. You *control* how you respond and what you do. You *cooperate,* both with others and with your own aims and desires. And that may require *compromise* (but only of a sort that doesn't deny the truth of who you are or what you feel).

The three C's were missing in the modeling that Roy got as a boy and young man. But the power tools can teach him control, cooperation, and compromise. And they can help you too; they *will* help you, if you use them. By getting yourself back, you get the ability to give and take with others, and be in relationships with others and the world around you. But it requires that you acknowledge and honor the inner reality, which is, "This isn't feeling good to me."

Looking Ahead

Throughout the rest of this book, we'll look at a variety of emotions and the behaviors they produce. We'll examine the development and existence of conflicts on the various levels of inner reality. In each case we'll also examine alternatives that are available to those who are willing to draw from their spiritual reality.

These alternatives are available to readers who are willing and ready to relinquish their dependency on what goes on *outside* them as the determinant of what goes on *inside* them. These alternatives are available to those who are willing to take responsibility for themselves and their lives, drawing from the rich soil of Spirit, as it lives within them, for the strength, power, and freedom that they desire and deserve.

Please know before we go any further that this isn't going to be easy. Relearning never is. Honoring internal commitments to oneself isn't easy either. Worthwhile, yes! Rewarding, absolutely! Easy to do—*get a grip!* But perhaps you'd already figured out that *easy* isn't the issue here—especially if you saw any part of yourself in Roy.

We've all been programmed to accept, embrace, and enact things about ourselves that aren't true. This doesn't necessarily mean that we believe them in our heart of hearts. It means simply that, although such assumptions may not be true, we defend them. We protect them with our thoughts, feelings, and beliefs about ourselves. Our defense is based on the fact that if we let go of what we think we know about ourselves, we won't have anything else to rely on.

The prospect of losing ourselves, even momentarily, can be pretty frightening. But that's what we have to do: we have to lose the false self to find the true one. The process of work presented in this book is about doing the hard, sometimes scary work associated with living your life from the inside out, so that in the end the *real you* can live a *real life*. This book will challenge you to live from the level of spiritual reality to the realm of physical manifestation, although we've all been taught to live the other way around. This work requires that you give up some long-held positions that have provided you with comfort and pleasure, in order to engage in a process designed to make you (and those who have supported you in being comfortable) *uncomfortable*. The premise is that when you're comfortable, you're not growing.

The work presented in this book is about growing—growing into your inherent power and experiencing the freedom of choice and expression that lies dormant therein. This work is about the self—self-awareness, self-development, self-care, self-empowerment, and self-support. *Self,* with a capital S, meaning the essence of divinity, meaning Spirit within you.

Therefore, this work is sacred work. It's secret work. Should it become very difficult for you, should you feel that you can't remain committed or that you're not seeing the results you desire, I encourage you in that moment to ask for help. Not from anyone or anything outside yourself, however. Rather, call forth the grace and power of Spirit within you. Ask, and you shall receive!

3

Phillip

Acting Up and Acting Out

It's one thing to be late. It's another thing altogether to be late *and to have an attitude*. Phillip arrived at the office, his attitude in tow, ten minutes late for a meeting he was scheduled to attend. He burst into the conference room about three minutes later. No one attending the meeting had any idea that Phillip had spent the night arguing with his girlfriend of three years. Nor did they know that he had just broken up with her for the fifth time in three years.

They knew that Phillip was upset about *something*—that much was evident—but no one asked for details, and Phillip didn't tell. No one at the meeting had any idea how to approach Phillip, given his attitude. He sat slouched down in his chair, a frown on his face. He doodled on the agenda as his colleagues talked. When it was his turn to report on his department, he rolled his eyes and said, "I'll pass." Then he flicked his pen across the table. His friend Gary caught it and slid it back toward him.

After the departmental reports, the manager moved on to the next item of business: the progress of employee teams. Unfortunately, he made the mistake of beginning with Phillip's team. No one can quite remember exactly what the manager said by way of introduction, but the consensus is that it was something about either attendance or lateness. Before the manager's words were fully formed and expressed, Phillip slammed his open palm on the table and vehemently denied what he apparently believed were accusations directed against him.

Ben, often the peacemaker in the group, jumped in, making a wholehearted effort to explain to Phillip exactly what the manager had been talking about, and how it related to him. Poor Ben! Either he had been sleeping, had been having an out-of-body experience, or just didn't care about Phillip or his attitude. In any case, the look that Phillip shot him could have sunk a ship. Beside Phillip, Mark saw the look and dropped his head so that he wouldn't have to see anything else.

The manager had a feeling that things were about to explode, so he asked Phillip to explain his position. Phillip, however, was dangerously focused on Ben, who was still trying to explain the manager's intentions. Whenever Ben started a sentence, Phillip interrupted with a counterargument. Pam, who was generally pretty good at helping her colleagues see an alternate point of view, interrupted to urge Phillip to listen to Ben's explanation. Elizabeth, too concerned about budget figures to get involved over what she saw as bickering over mundane matters, had tuned out and was adding numbers on her paper.

Still Ben kept talking. But suddenly Phillip was talking louder, and it was clear that things were coming to a head. No one knows who stood up first, Phillip or the manager. But it was Phillip who first took decisive action: before anyone could get a handle on the situation, he threw a chair across the table. It was aimed at Ben, but he threw himself to the floor and the chair sailed overhead to clatter against the wall. Then the chaos took on a life of its own. Suddenly Pam was on the table, the manager was smashed to the wall, and Elizabeth was heading for the door, calculator in hand. Gary rushed to hold on to Phillip, who was walking toward Ben with a look of pure malice.

When it was all over, no one had been hurt. The police weren't called. Phillip apologized. Ben accepted. The manager typed up a letter of termination for Phillip to submit, but before he could deliver it to Mr. Attitude, Phillip had packed up his desk and left.

The first call Phillip made once he got home was to his girlfriend. When she heard what had happened, she forgot that they were fighting and took his side. The next call Phillip made was to his best friend, who was working on a project but promised to call him later. It wasn't until he called his mother that he heard the truth: "I guess you acted up and acted out one time too many," she said. "*Now* what are you going to do?"

What's Really Going On?

I grew up in Brooklyn, New York, where I watched my brother and a wide circle of his friends struggle through the complexities associated with young boys growing into men. Much of what I saw and overheard had no meaning whatsoever to me, as a flat-chested, insecure hormonal hotbed. My brother and his friends spoke another language than what I used with my circle of female friends. A language of few words, with obviously deep (though symbolic) meanings.

The symbols and the language became most apparent

whenever a new guy attempted to join the ranks. It was then that I saw how the group sniffed him out, challenged him verbally and nonverbally, as a way of determining whether or not he was who he claimed to be. It was then, when a new guy came around, that I caught glimpses of the differences between males and females. Everything seemed to hang on the language—that verbal and nonverbal language which carried deeply profound messages that only "the guys" understood.

There was one spoken challenge in particular that seemed to have a great deal of significance to a new guy who broke rank. It was something like, "Don't let your mouth write a check that your butt can't cash." For the life of me, I couldn't figure out why football-loving cardplayers would use banking and financial issues as a foundation for ritualistic acceptance into the group!

When you allow your pride, ego, or pain to motivate your speech or behavior in regard to another person, you're writing a check, so to speak. How so? Well, you're setting up a medium of exchange that will eventually become the foundation for the relationship being negotiated between yourself and that other person.

When you write that check to someone who plays a significant role in your well-being or survival, the negotiations can be extremely difficult. The negotiations are more challenging still when you enter into them with wounded pride, an unchecked ego, or a conscious or unconscious emotional wound. Under those circumstances, chances are you'll say or do something that will create a serious deficit in some aspect of your life.

The person with whom you're in negotiations will more likely than not be unable or unwilling to cash the emotional check you've written. Not because he or she doesn't *want* to cash it, but because of the way you present it. This dynamic happens all the time between parents and children.

It's important to understand where we learned how to present our checks, because the relationships we establish with our parents or childhood caregivers generally serve as the foundation for our later *emotional negotiation skills*. These skills create our *inner reality*—the reality from which we live and conduct our lives.

Although I say "inner reality" in the singular, each of us lives under the constant influence of four distinctly separate but interrelated inner realities: physical reality, mental reality, emotional reality, and spiritual reality. Let's look at each of these in turn.

Physical Reality

Physical reality is a function of that which we can see, feel, hear, touch, and taste; in other words, it's the reality of the physical senses. This level is crucial to human life.

It's at the level of physical reality within our being, and related to our environment, that we learn to *seek pleasure* and, at all costs, *avoid pain*. It's at the level of physical reality that, as children, we learn to enjoy what feels good and to avoid what doesn't.

We learn to experiment with and create boundaries, learning how far we can go and what we can do before the pleasure stops and the pain begins. We learn how far we can go before someone screams at us or swats us on the behind. We learn who swats the hardest, and who will attach a kiss or hug to a swat. We learn which holes we can stick our fingers into, and which holes are off-limits. We learn that the brown stuff wrapped in paper is sweet and the green stuff on the plate is nasty! We learn about safety, security, and hiding from what is or isn't safe. More important, we learn who and what to trust to increase our pleasure, and who and what will and won't inflict pain.

Our physical reality is powerfully linked to, and translated by, our inner mental reality, which we turn to next.

Mental Reality

Mental reality is the storehouse of our memories, our past experiences. At the level of this inner reality, we store what we've learned from experience, what we've been taught by those who provide care and guidance, and what we perceive or hold to be true based on that learning and experience.

It's at the mental level of our inner reality that we figure out more generally, to the best of our ability, what's pleasurable and what's painful. We make associations, moving from what we actually know to what we expect based on that knowledge. At the level of mental reality we step beyond the stage of experimentation in the memory of the senses—the stage grounded in physical reality—which may or may not be accurate in all situations. We gradually come to *believe,* based on the mental associations we create, that we have *concrete evidence* as to what's painful and what's pleasurable; who can and will inflict pain or increase pleasure; how to avoid, negotiate, or eliminate pain; and how to transform pain into pleasure.

In the midst of our learning at the level of mental reality, we're also creating the learning tools of our emotional reality.

Emotional Reality

No matter how you cut it, or who you are, we all have a common goal in life: do what feels good and avoid what doesn't! While there may be supportive evidence for our physical and mental realities, our emotional reality is purely subjective. It exists within us based on what we think, what we know, and how we feel.

Emotional reality is powerful because it provides the evidence of what we experience on the physical level, while it intensifies what we perceive on the mental level. It determines what we do, and how we do it, in response to the stimuli encountered at the other two levels. The stimuli create what I call an *emotional charge.* The charge we get from a particular experience or stimulation will either propel us forward or hold us back.

We can't move at all if our heart, our emotional reality, isn't invested in what we're doing. The emotions, more than any other aspect of our being, determine our responses, actions, reactions, and ability to negotiate through our experiences. Our emotional reality is the clean-burning fuel of our lives.

Thoughts are fuel too, as are memories. Associations, beliefs, and perceptions all serve as fuel—but not all of them burn equally well. Unfortunately, when we mix good fuel with bad fuel, real fuel with cheap impostors, the vehicle we're driving can break down, leaving us stuck!

Spiritual Reality

Beneath the physical, mental, and emotional realities, there's much more fertile ground. This is the *inner spiritual reality.* The authentic reality. The truth of who we are. It's here that the spark and essence of divinity have been embedded in our being. This is the real fuel tank. It's the mother lode! It's what's been called the still small voice. The glimmer of hope. The spark of genius that shines through our eyes, inspiring thought and flooding the heart with possibilities.

It's from this inner spiritual level that we're meant to live. It's from this inner spiritual reality that we're empowered to create and live full and abundant lives. It's from this level that we get the strength and courage to put up with and live through all that we encounter and experience at the other levels of reality. This is the level of our being at which we discover and experience freedom. Freedom of thought. Freedom of expression. Freedom of movement to negotiate the inner and outer realities that we desire to experience.

And yet it's this level of pure divine essence that we're

taught, trained, programmed, and encouraged to *ignore*. In the process, we become mentally confused, emotionally conflicted, and tragically disarmed and disabled at the level of our physical reality.

Knowing this, let's take another look at Phillip.

Talking to the Man in the Mirror

Phillip is a man. Like all men, he was trained to do certain kinds of things. He's expected to do them. In doing these manly things, there's an inner urge to experience pleasure and avoid pain. At first glance, it makes perfectly good sense: Phillip wants to feel good about *himself* while he's doing what makes him feel good as a *man*. This is the physical reality in which we all live.

Whether or not Phillip was *taught* how to do what men do, he was certainly *trained,* by experience and/or example, to do what men do; and this training, coupled with his perceived ability to meet the criteria of both the inner and outer expectations, undergirds Phillip's mental reality. What he thinks about himself (and his ability to do what men do) and what he thinks *others* think about him collide at the point of the *doing*.

Next we must consider Phillip's primary fuel source: his emotions. When we meet Phillip, suffice it to say he's a tad bit upset. He's been fighting with his girlfriend. If she's worth her weight in womanliness, she probably said some pretty ugly and hurtful things to Phillip. We can also venture to guess that Phillip has perceived some of the things she said as a frontal attack on his manhood. Chances are she made him feel *wrong,* pointing out all the *wrong* things he did or said.

If Phillip is anything like 99.9 percent of the rest of the human race, wrong is bad! It's even worse when you're a man, though, because men are punished severely for doing wrong: their women lose hope, faith, and trust in them, and their peers look disapprovingly at them. This isn't a new lesson for Phillip, of course. He learned it when he first stuck his finger in the wrong socket as a toddler, and he reviewed it every time he cried over a skinned knee or missed a catch on the football field.

Now, scrolling back to adulthood, couple the anger of Phillip's girlfriend with the fact that Phillip is late for an important meeting at work. The straws are piling up on the camel's back: he's doing *something else* wrong; he's *bad!* And as Phillip has learned, there's absolutely no pleasure in being bad. Can you imagine the train wreck going on in Phillip's head? It's called conflict. And the combination of mental and emotional conflict equals pain!

In the midst of Phillip's painful conflict, there's something that he—*the man*—is expected to do. He has to earn a living! He has to go to work! Men *must* work, no matter how they feel on the inside. Men are expected to suspend their inner reality (if need be) in order to meet the outward expectations that have been placed on them, or that they've placed on themselves. It's expected that men will *handle or hide* what they feel in order to do what's expected of them.

Phillip no doubt wanted, at the height of the argument with his girlfriend, to convince her that he wasn't wrong, *but he had to go to work!* His mental images of manhood were urging him to avenge the perceived attack made by his girlfriend on his manhood, *but he had to go to work!* Phillip the pleasure-seeker wanted to be comforted, to experience a brief moment of reassurance, *but he had to go to work!* After all, at his place of employment there were people waiting for him, *depending* on him, *expecting* that he would show up and do what men do. Work! *Oh, the inhumanity!*

How is a human being supposed to negotiate the troubled waters of his own inner reality while experiencing conflict and pain with the outer ones—and all this when he's running on cheap fuel and tainted memories? Beats the heck out of me, but we do it all the time—men and women alike! We ignore, avoid, deny, and compromise what we're experiencing inwardly in order to meet outward expectations. Though this human tendency knows no gender, it's much more tragic for men. Why? Because men don't cry. Because, with rare exceptions, men don't have close, intimate, and honest associations with other men on whom they can lean and depend. Because men don't lean; men don't depend!

What men do when there's a mental or emotional train wreck going on inside themselves is *act out*. Acting out is an indirect and generally unconscious way of engaging patterns of conflict, pain, or dysfunction. Men who act out may feel better in the short term, but the relief is only temporary, because the underlying conflict remains unresolved. In the long term, acting out re-creates the very sort of experiences it aims to avoid, reinforcing the physical, mental, and emotional realities that created the conflict and pain in the first place!

Which brings us back to Phillip. As he storms late into the office, he's fuming over the fact that he isn't being heard. It seems to him that his girlfriend simply can't hear what he's trying to say. He knows the feeling well, because he wasn't heard as a child either. And it's not a good feeling. When people feel that they aren't being heard, they often experience a sense of worthlessness. They conclude, "Who I am, what I say, what I need doesn't matter."

Phillip is also experiencing fear. He's afraid that he's done the wrong thing, in the wrong way—which, as we've seen, is easily perceived and translated as "I'm bad!" Furthermore, Phillip is afraid of being punished for being bad. He probably associates the difficult experience with his girlfriend with some latent, unconscious memory of a childhood crime and punishment. Because of that association, he now fears that since he's been bad, he'll lose a source of pleasure, comfort, and reassurance.

Losing is *never* pleasurable! It's a powerful mental and emotional trigger for us all, but *especially* for men. The concepts of winning and losing are intricately tied to manhood and manliness. It must be all of those sports competitions and locker room discussions!

Most important, Phillip is angry. Anger is a mental and emotional response to having our inherent sense of power ignored, diminished, or taken away. Phillip can't make his girlfriend hear him. He can't convince her that he's right. He perceives that she's ignoring his power, while at the same time he can't seem to activate or utilize the power that he knows he has. If only she'd *listen!* If only he could *make* her hear him! If only he could eliminate the pain of the mental and emotional conflict and experience a moment of pleasure.

Phillip doesn't know it, but if he could reach beyond the programming, training, and past experiences, down into the rich soil of his spirit, he would find another alternative. Unfortunately, he doesn't know he even *has* a spirit. What's more, he has to go to work! And he's late!

Sleeping Dogs Don't Sleep Forever!

Every thought that has ever crossed through our brains; every emotion, pleasurable or not; every perception, judgment, learning, and association from every experience, training, or programming we've ever received—all these are lying dormant within our being. Some of them bark. Some of them bite. Some of them whimper. But they all play a role in why and how we do what we do. We feed these dogs moment by moment with every new thought, emotion, expectation, belief, association, action, and interaction. We feed them with our inner realities of mind, emotion, and spirit, but they're simultaneously being fed with the outer reality in which we find ourselves. Food is fuel! The nature of the fuel of our combined inner and outer realities determines whether we're raising a vicious pit bull or a timid spaniel.

Fear is a pit bull! When you are in fear—the fear of not being heard, not being acknowledged, or the fear that *who you are* and *what you feel* is unworthy—any checks you write will be scripted by your wounded pride. Some inner aspect of your being will be screaming out in your brain, "That person thinks I'm a pushover!" In the worst-case scenario, the prideful voice in the back of your mind will taunt you: "Just who does she think she is? She can't treat me like this! I'll show her who I am!" In other cases your pride may be silent, telling you nothing at all. No clear direction. No guidance about what to do next. No inner support or validation. This silence is probably more frightening than being taunted or goaded into action.

Whether you hear a message or not, when you're in the grip of fear, the ego becomes your mental and emotional checkwriter. The ego, that dark-winged angel who often whispers conflicting messages to you, will bring to the forefront of your thinking every embarrassing, humiliating, dishonorable past experience it can conjure up in thirty seconds or less. Like a rabid dog, it will remind you of every unkind experience you've ever had. The memory of everyone who's ever challenged you, or made fun of your name, or hit you harder than you could hit them will wake up and start barking.

When wounded pride and an unchecked ego are negotiating on your behalf, you will remember every relay race you ever lost. Every spelling test you ever failed. Right before your eyes will flash that one long-ago incident when he was really, really afraid or really, really unsure of himself and reached out for help, only to be laughed at, abandoned, rejected, or not even heard. It's that memory in particular that's going to bring the energy up from the pit of the man's stomach, via his testosterone, straight into his brain, causing him to act up or act out.

In response to a dog barking in the brain, you may become violent, or you may shut down. In either case, anyone who comes into contact with you will also meet the dog face-to-face, because your behavior will be a reflection of how that inner dog has been trained to behave. You growl, bark, snap, bite, or run away, depending on what that barking internal dog tells you to do.

In most cases, a man who's been trained or programmed by experience or example about the manly thing to do when confronted by a dog won't run away. Instead, he'll defend himself. *How* he defends himself is a function of his inner reality, the number and breeds of dogs that come alive in his consciousness.

In Phillips's case, the pit bull woke up, growled, barked, and caused him to bite. Biting is a form of acting out—one form among many. War is another way of acting out. Alcoholism, substance abuse, and barroom brawls, while not limited to the domain of males, are common ways in which men act *up* and act *out*.

Men typically act out when they feel powerless, oppressed, afraid, or angry. They also act out when there's a conflict among the levels of their inner reality. Men tend to act out when they're in pain. This isn't an excuse. It is, however, a reality that most of us live with.

Activating Spiritual Energy

The human psyche can take only so much before it seeks an outlet from pain or conflict. It seeks out the most accessible source of release, relying on habits, expressions, and outlets that it believes will assuage the pain. Unfortunately, in the process of finding relief, the human psyche often draws from the very level of inner reality—whether the physical, mental, or emotional level—that's the source of the pain or conflict. In other words, it seeks to both draw energy from and release energy to the same level of reality. That's like cutting off your nose to spite your face!

There's another level of reality, as we saw earlier: the spiritual level. And because that level is the fuel tank, an inexhaustible amount of energy can be drawn from it. Furthermore, the energy drawn from this level is transformational; it facilitates change. The outer conditions, situations, and experiences don't change. Rather, change occurs within, on all levels of the inner reality.

The question is, *How?* How do you activate spiritual energy in the midst of painful internal conflict? The answer is, *Process*. In order to access and activate spiritual energy, you must be willing to engage in the process of moving your humanness out of the way and allowing the energy of your divinity—your spirit, which is part of the divine Spirit—to take over. You must be willing to live within a process of checking in with yourself, checking up on yourself, and supporting yourself by applying spiritual principles to your thoughts and feelings.

The good news is, no one has to know what you're doing. The spiritual process takes place in the inner, unseen realms of your being. The bad news is, you're 100 percent responsible for working through the process. Whether or not the process works for you is dependent entirely on your efforts. Unlike the physical, mental, and emotional levels of reality, you can't get away with leaving little things undone on the spiritual level. You either work the process, or you don't. You either take the steps, one at a time, to bring your inner reality into balance, or you don't. You either take responsibility for what you think, what you feel, and how you behave in response to your thoughts and feelings, or you don't. If you start the process of using spiritual energy as a way to resolve conflict, and then you stop, the conflict will remain and the pain may intensify. And if you're aware that the spiritual process is a viable alternative but choose not to employ it at all, both the conflict and the pain will *certainly* intensify.

One of the main reasons men rarely draw on their spiritual energy as a way to resolve painful inner conflict is that *they haven't been taught how*. We're not talking here about taking a few moments to pray or taking a few deep breaths. These things help, of course, but they only scratch the surface. In fact, many men will do just that—breathe, pray, and call themselves spiritual. I call this approach the "spiritual bypass." It's a function of mouthing spiritual principles, using spiritual concepts, but continuing to act from the pit of the human ego and consciousness.

In learning to live from the level of your own inner spiritual reality, you must know and be willing to employ *spiritual principles*. Spiritual principles are the keys to transforming reality at the physical, mental, and emotional levels. Spiritual principles are at the heart of the power tools presented here, and they'll give you the strength, courage, and insight to *unlearn* what you've been taught as you *relearn* the truth of your authentic self, your spiritual self.

Men like tools. Tools can be used to create, build, tear down, and rebuild. Spiritual principles, when used as tools, can help us do all these things. They support us in creating a new reality, a new way of being, by offering us a process and system for building. They also help with the preliminary work of tearing down old structures and paradigms and rebuilding what's salvageable.

Because spiritual principles allow us to rebuild a structure from which and through which we can live more peacefully, abundantly, and powerfully, they're the keys to freedom. They free us from the prison walls that we've erected in our hearts and minds in response to programming, conditioning, experience, and observation. They set us free from the limitations we've erected in our physical reality out of loyalty to the teaching, training, perceptions, judgments, and beliefs of those who loved us enough to teach us *what they knew* in an attempt to spare us the pain and conflict they experienced in their own lives. They give us the power to tear down all the concepts and constructs that created (and still contribute to) the pain and conflict we experience, and to rebuild a life from inside our being.

Unfortunately, Phillip, like most of us, didn't know that this alternative existed for him. He didn't know what to do or how to do it. Let's examine what might have happened had he known.

Phillip was angry. Anger usually explodes. Phillip was angry because for most of his life, he *felt* as if he had not been heard. In his early years, he thought his father didn't care enough to listen and his mother was too busy to listen. When Phillip wanted to get his parents' attention, he couldn't just speak up; he had to act out. When he did, they'd stop and take notice. By then, though, it was too late: their attention was focused on *what he had done,* how he had acted out, rather than on what it was he'd been trying to say by acting out. It was, however, the only way Phillip knew to get his parents to listen to what he had to say.

As he grew older, he used the same strategy in his relationships. When Phillip felt that a friend or a girlfriend or co-worker wasn't listening or couldn't hear what he was saying, he acted out. He threw things, he broke things in an attempt to get his point across. In all other respects, though, Phillip was a sweet guy, which is probably why people put up with that kind of crap from him.

Beneath the anger of not being heard, Phillip harbored the belief that *he didn't matter.* Although there was a part of him, something inside of him, that knew it wasn't really true, that something wasn't enough to sustain him when he felt the anger rising up his spine. After all, he continued to encounter evidence in his physical reality that he didn't matter to the people who mattered to him. That really ticked him off! What he *thought* didn't matter—obviously, since people didn't listen to him. What he *felt* didn't matter—same reason. On bad days, he went so far as to believe that what he *did* and how he did it didn't matter. He *thought* his unworth, he *felt* it, and he *believed* it.

Despite the fact that these were *his* thoughts, *his* feelings, and *his* beliefs, Phillip made everyone else responsible for them. This is a reflection of the danger we all encounter when we're left alone in our own heads without the proper tools. Phillip didn't see that although the people around him reinforced his thoughts, feelings, and beliefs by responding (as his friends and colleagues did) to his acting out, the thoughts, feelings, and beliefs were his to begin with, and they remain his. He needs to take responsibility for them.

Phillip seemed helpless to do that. He knew that there was a major conflict between what he did and who he believed himself to be. He knew that his behavior was often neither appropriate nor acceptable. And yet, in the moments when he experienced the intensity of an inner conflict or the intensity of his anger, he resorted to acting out because he'd learned through experience that it always worked to get him what he wanted: to be heard and to matter.

The spiritual principle, the power tool that Phillip needs most, is *responsibility*. Only if he masters that tool will he understand that he has a *choice* in what he does; only then will he understand that what he chooses to do, he can choose *not* to do.

Phillip must learn to take responsibility for his own thoughts and feelings: what he *thinks* others think and feel about him is his responsibility; what he *feels* in response to what he thinks others think and feel is also his responsibility. But Phillip must also learn to take responsibility to ensure that he's heard. Men who believe that they're generally not being heard often don't say anything about things that they deem important because they *assume* that no one will listen. That's a habit that starts when they're children. By the time they reach adulthood, they expect people to read their mind. They expect others to know what they mean, deduce what they want, figure out what they're trying to say—even when they say nothing at all!

Here's how taking responsibility in this area might look. When Phillip has something to say, he needs to make sure first that he actually says it. That's easier said than done for someone used to holding his tongue. It may be as simple as saying, "I've got something to say." Or, "I need to say something." Once he has spoken, it is Phillip's responsibility to check in with the other person, making sure that what he has said has been heard. This doesn't mean that the other person must agree with, or even accept, what Phillip has said. It means that it is Phillip's responsibility to deliver the message.

Taking responsibility in this area is important because, as Phillip knows well, *delivery* and *receipt* aren't the same thing. But he needs to remember that *receipt* and *agreement* are likewise two different beasts. Chances are, since Phillip has convinced himself that he isn't being heard and that he doesn't matter, any disagreement he encounters will evoke anger; and in Phillip's life, anger is a motivator for acting out. Taking responsibility for his choices will support Phillip in unlearning this pattern of behavior.

I mentioned earlier that responsibility is closely linked to choice. How Phillip responds to his own belief that he isn't being heard is a function of choice. All behaviors, responses, and reactions happen as the result of choice. Oh sure, we'd all like to believe that there are instances when we have no choice in how we behave. Unfortunately, this is *never* true. There are times when the moment between choice and action is so brief—for example, when we believe we're in danger—that we don't realize we're making a choice. We believe that our responses are involuntary. Yet the truth is, we're always *choosing* how to behave, how to respond. The body can't volunteer to do anything without clear direction from the mind. And mental direction is a choice.

Supporting us in our choices are the parameters and elements of our mental and emotional realities, as well as the physical reality of our environment. Phillip learned that by acting out, he could get someone to listen to him. Because acting out worked, he chose it as his primary mode of communication. Phillip made this his behavior of choice.

Phillip's transformation plan (willingness, readiness, and ability), the process of using the spiritual tools of choice and responsibility, would look something like this.

Transformation Plan and Power Tools

What would it take to get Phillip to change? A lot! But it can be done if he uses the power tools of awareness, acknowledgment, responsibility—Phillip's biggie—forgiveness, and commitment.

Awareness

Phillip needs to spend time with himself, becoming aware of both his mental reality and his emotional reality. Having done that, he then has to examine all of the elements that have *contributed* to his mental and emotional realities. Only if he's aware of his inner workings will he be able to change them.

Acknowledgment

Acknowledgment is an essential tool in Phillip's transformation process. Once he becomes aware of his mental and emotional realities, he needs to see them, acknowledging to himself every time he has the impulse to hide or act out. He needs to do this on a daily basis, not only in regard to his job or his relationship but in all areas of his life. Keeping a daily journal is one way he might accomplish this goal. Therapy is another.

Making himself aware of the elements that have contributed to his mental and emotional realities—parents, siblings, peers, teachers, experiences, and so on—may involve revisiting some painful memories for the purpose of reinterpreting or releasing them.

Responsibility

Phillip needs to take full responsibility for how he's allowed his thoughts and feelings to motivate his actions. At this stage it's easy to fall into the trap of blaming other people, which is the exact opposite of taking responsibility. Taking responsibility means acknowledging "I did this because I felt that . . . ," or "When I thought that, I did this. . . ." Again, journal-writing is an excellent private and painless method for accomplishing this task.

Forgiveness

Phillip must be willing to forgive himself for choices he's made and actions he's taken that have caused harm to himself or others. This forgiveness is a sign that he's taking responsibility for his own actions. He must also be willing to forgive himself for the judgments he's held about or against himself, as well as those he's held about and against others. (A judgment is any thought or emotion that supports a person in holding the position that he or another person is bad or wrong.) Like Phillip, we're all responding to our inner realities. If our responses get us into trouble, it doesn't mean we're either bad or wrong. It simply means that we must learn how to respond from a different level of reality. Whether or not we learn to do so is a function of our willingness to *accept responsibility* for our own inner realities.

Once he's forgiven himself, Phillip will be able to get clear about what it is that he wants for himself, how he wants to handle himself, and how he wants to experience himself being in the world.

Commitment

Once he's forgiven himself, Phillip must get clear about what it is that he wants for himself and what he's willing and ready to do to clean up his act. If he wants to be heard, Phillip must make a commitment to speak up and check in to make sure that his message was both delivered and received. He must make a commitment to himself about how he'll channel his anger in a way that's more constructive than acting out. He must make a commitment to experience himself as a nice guy who can handle his own anger, who can keep himself in check, who can be peaceful, loving, and respectful no matter what anyone else says or does.

Once that commitment has been made, Phillip must honor it. He must draft a plan of action for channeling his anger so that he has recourse when he feels as if he isn't being heard. He must develop an effective way to remind himself that he does matter. The key, again, is responsibility: Phillip must take responsibility for keeping himself on track toward his commitment, regardless of the words and behavior of those around him.

Knowledge Equals the Freedom to Choose

None of the things in Phillip's transformation plan is easy, but all of them are definitely doable! Practice makes perfect; repetition is the mother of skill. If Phillip keeps his commitment to be engaged in the process of using spiritual principles as tools, and if he consistently practices the steps of the process, he will experience a shift within his being that will provide him with a variety of alternatives to acting out. The grace of Spirit will bring them into his consciousness, at which point he can choose what to do.

Unfortunately, a transformation plan is rarely a one-shot deal. Even if Phillip decides to attempt a transformation, he may well stumble along his path toward change. If and when he misses a step, if and when his old pattern of acting out reemerges, he'll have to rework his plan and his process. That's his responsibility too.

In order to live from the inner spiritual reality, we all face the same challenge Phillip does: we have to be willing to get off our current position. We have to be ready for and committed to taking responsibility for what goes on inside us. Once we make the commitment and set the intention to do the work of embracing a spiritual process, we need to become aware of everything we do. That's how the relearning takes place. As we become aware, we're empowered to make different, and hopefully *better,* choices. As our choices change, so will our experience of self and others.

Unfortunately, when it came right down to it, Phillip was neither willing nor ready to adopt a transformation plan and begin the work of rehabilitation. Though his girlfriend urged him to mend his ways, he claimed that his old memories were too painful to look at. His behavior, he said, was too ingrained to change. He took the "This is just how I am!" route, blaming others, allowing them to bear the weight of responsibility for his thoughts and feelings. He promised, though—as he had done repeatedly over the years—to try to control himself.

And because those others in Phillip's life loved him, they questioned themselves and accepted the responsibility. His girlfriend took him back, promising not to call him any more names. His best friend helped him find a new job, begging him not to embarrass him again. His mother made his bad behavior about *her,* saying that she should have punished him more when he was younger. In the end no one heard what Phillip was saying because no one could get past his *behavior* to his underlying *message*.

But perhaps that's not the end for Phillip. Maybe the next time he acts out in response to a serious conflict, he'll feel a pain severe enough to bring him to a willingness to change. If so, the power tools will help bring him to spiritual health and wholeness.

4

Eddie

Building Spiritual Muscle

Given the choice, Eddie would do something for you before he'd do it for himself. His motto has always been "selfless service"; his life, ever since childhood, has been built around doing good things for other people. That's how he gets his sense of value and worth: taking care of other people.

When it came time to choose a profession, Eddie decided to become a teacher. Later, he did some more coursework and became a beloved high school guidance counselor. Still in that job now, he's always solving problems for other people. Eddie is a very generous, loving, caring person. His worst fault is that he's never learned how to take care of his own needs.

On the surface, Eddie is a saint—the kind of guy mothers

love. But Eddie grew up in a home with no joy. His mother, who worked all the time, was too tired to deal with her family in anything other than a cursory way. Love was a luxury she couldn't afford. And his father? Absent. Walked out one day when Eddie was eight, promising he'd be back. Eddie and his older brother and younger sister are still waiting.

Eddie is staring down the barrel of his fiftieth birthday, and he's spending a lot of time looking back over his life. He's on his third marriage, and it's more than a little rocky. He has four kids; two are college graduates, and all of them are getting on with their own lives. His oldest son is married and building his own family. Eddie is seeing his kids make many of the same mistakes he did when he was younger, though, and that hurts. Most of them are in and out of relationships, just as he's been. It makes him sad.

His longest marriage has been to wife number three. Also an educator, she was a high school teacher when they met. But lately, almost without Eddie realizing what happened, his wife has swept past him in terms of both financial and professional accomplishments. He hardly noticed when she was first elected to the local school board. He didn't even pay much heed when she was chosen to *head* that group. But it was hard to miss the attention (or the proposed honorarium) when she was appointed by the governor to a special task force on education. There she was on TV and in the papers.

The day after her appointment, a front-page article in their hometown paper noted that she was married to a guidance counselor. A guidance counselor? That's what he was. That's *all* he was: the economically inferior, less accomplished spouse of a now high-powered, high-profile woman, also a professional educator, who had accomplished a great deal more financial and professional success than he has doing the same kind of work. Lately she has begun challenging him about taking care of himself. And now she's been appointed by the governor to a special advisory position created to look at education in the state and make some recommendations. All of a sudden his wife's in the news. All of a sudden his wife is making serious money. She just testified before Congress in a televised session. This has brought Eddie to a state of crisis.

Eddie's wife has come back from Washington, D.C., and she's saying that he isn't contributing enough financially. He doesn't have an adequate wardrobe. He drives a raggedy car. She's creating a college fund for her grandchildren, and he has nothing to offer his. And he's using the resources that she's bringing to the relationship to take care of himself.

Eddie has never felt that he is in competition with his wife, but suddenly he finds himself going up against her. And losing. The truth is, he *is* dependent on her, both financially and emotionally. He *does* need her on every level.

So instead of dealing with that, he starts in on her. "All this work, this travel, this testifying in Washington is destroying our relationship," he says plaintively.

"How so?" she asks.

That's all the opening he needs. He becomes critical and judgmental and starts to tear her down. "You're never here," he complains. "You don't care anymore. All you want is power. You've forgotten about service."

This conclusion doesn't do much for his wife, who sees his envy more clearly than he does and who wouldn't mind a little recognition of her own. Hell, she's worked for it. "You could do it too, if you'd get off your ass," she says, a little more sharply than she'd intended.

"No, I couldn't," he counters. "You got your appointment because you're a woman."

And back and forth it goes, and soon there's a crisis in his marriage, sure enough.

But it's not only his marriage that's causing Eddie pain. It's hard for him to watch his children struggle in their own lives, in their own relationships. They're all asking him for support and help that he can't give them. His eldest son needs some support in getting his first house, and Eddie doesn't have any money to spare; his youngest daughter is in turmoil over a guy she's dating, and he can't seem to muster up any advice. After all these years of helping everybody in the world, after all these years of helping everybody else's children, he can't even help his own! It hurts to admit it, but he has nothing to offer them—financially, emotionally, professionally.

What does he do? He makes his wife wrong; *she's* the bad guy. What comes out of his mouth is criticism, when what's really going on inside him is "I'm not as good as you are," and "How come when we're doing the same thing, you're moving forward and I'm not?" Though he knows at some level that she's not to blame, he tries to make it all her fault; and in his anger at his lack of perceived manliness, he becomes passive-aggressive.

Talking to the Man in the Mirror

Eddie reminds me of my ex-husband, who wasn't a bad person but who had some very bad habits. Among these, the most damaging were negative self-talk, expecting the worst, people-pleasing, seeking validation from an external source (usually other people), and blaming others for what he couldn't do in life.

He learned these habits in an environment that didn't support his true inner identity but instead judged him by what he did and by what others thought of him. He learned these habits in a home where his mother intimidated him into submission (passing on her fear that unless he was submissive, he would fail in life). He learned them in an educational system that was grounded in historical distortion and blatant dishonesty.

The driving force in each of these environments was control. I believe that our human institutions are designed to control the minds of people and the inherent nature of men. Despite the conflict between what my husband felt and what the world demanded of him, he—like so many Black men—tried to acquire the sense of power that society told him he must have as a man. Unfortunately, that same society forgot to tell him that his *real* power lay dormant in his soul.

Eddie faces a similar problem. In this world where we confuse our true nature—our "who"—with our occupation—our "do"—men like Eddie and my ex-husband get lost. Eddie has lost his identity, his spiritual empowerment. Because he's lived his life getting his power not from his spiritual being but from taking care of others, when it comes time to take care of himself he's all out of whack—no balance, no sense of worth.

The problem becomes clearer when we realize that Eddie cares for others over himself because at a deep, central level he doesn't feel that he *deserves* care; he doesn't think that he's *worthy*. Maybe it's because his father promised to come back and didn't; maybe it's because his mother was too busy to get to know him. How and why it happened doesn't really matter now that he's almost fifty. What *does* matter is that he's spent his whole life giving to others what no one, himself included, has been able to give to him.

Not that no one tried. A few people—including his wives—did, but he turned them down. He thanked them and told them that he didn't need any help. He was fine; he had what he needed; thanks but no thanks.

And now, as he's assessing his life (past and present), his conclusion is that he's given that life over to other people and has nothing to show for it. That conclusion makes him angry. Sad too. Very, very sad.

It's not that he's underachieved; quite the contrary. It's not that he hasn't worked hard and to good effect. It's not that he doesn't feel that what he's done with his life is worthy. It's that *he* doesn't feel worthy. Not for lack of trying, though: in fact, he's worked so hard to feel worthy that he's exhausted himself.

Eddie's problem is a lack of balance between the inner and the outer, the spiritual and the material, the true power and powerlessness. That same issue is at the center of the problem of most men.

I remember one morning about ten years ago. It was Thanksgiving, and I awakened at 6:20 A.M. with a jolt. What woke me was the kind of spiritual experience to which I'd become accustomed during the years of my journey. I still had a lot of cooking to do, but this jolt wasn't about turkey and dressing. It was a spiritual calling.

When the jolt hit, it was sharp but imprecise. Not knowing what I was being called to do, I sat straight up, threw my legs over the side of the bed, and began my usual morning prayer of thanksgiving. Then suddenly it hit me like a thunderbolt: *Write a book for the spiritual empowerment of Black men.* This wasn't the first time that thought had occurred to me. But now it was compelling.

I wasn't about to just say yes, though. I asked, "Why me?"—my usual question when prompted by Spirit to do what seems impossible. The answer came back loud and clear: *Balance.* Everything in life must be balanced. What I do for and give to women, I realized, I had to do for and give to men.

That ten-year-old truth has never been truer. All of us, women as much as men, have fallen out of balance, just as Eddie has. Men have fallen *out* of their hearts into their heads. Women have fallen *over* their hearts into their heads. We've all fallen out of the grace of Spirit. We've been conditioned to honor a system of values built on contempt and disrespect for who we are as a community of people.

As a result of our fall, we're in conflict with both the value system of the society in which we live and our own basic nature. Men who instinctively want to stand among the leaders and direct the tides of the living world often sit in fear of being hung out to dry (and left hanging) or annihilated. Women who want to stand by or stand up for their male counterparts are often stepped on or stepped over, accused by the very ones they desire to support of being out of "their place" and attempting to take over. Although our basic nature is to embrace and support each other while taking the necessary steps toward a collective goal, we've been conditioned to compete with and against each other. We now treat each other as adversaries rather than allies.

In all honesty, I, for one, have been able to identify many

ways and times I have been guilty of this divisive behavior. Men and women struggle to understand and balance our gender roles at home, at work, and within a context of social responsibilities, while many of us are at a total loss as to how to balance our *individual* physical, emotional, and spiritual needs and responsibilities.

The instinctual nature of the woman is to give and share, yet our conditioning encourages us to see usury and manipulation around every corner. While men love to be cared for and nurtured by women, social programming makes men suspicious that caring women are trying to take over, take control. The basic human instinct to be loving and caring is often overshadowed by ego needs, image-building, and peer pressure. While Mama and Daddy preach, "Do unto others" and "Love thy neighbor," the world teaches us, "Everyone for himself when we hit the beach!" Fear of losing ground has replaced faith. The urge to give unselfishly has been overshadowed by the compulsion to get. Rather than using things to help and serve people, we follow society's teaching and use people to get things. In the process, we lose a vital piece of our spiritual soul. Restoration of what we've lost, rebalancing of the imbalance that we feel, is critical for all of us—especially, though, for men.

In the spiritual universe, we have approached a critical time. This is a time when the spiritual energy and role of the male is quickly changing, desperately needed, and sorely missed. Men must shine again. Be warm again. Stand in the face of the woman without fear, anger, or the need to hold on to a competitive edge. The major goal is to begin the process of recognition, alignment, in honor of men among yourselves.

I've tried to do what I could to correct the fact that not enough is being done to provide men with the truth about their spiritual identity, the truth of who we are at the core of our being. Spirituality is the consciously active means by which we can recognize, activate, and live the impartial, non-judgmental, consistent truth of who we are.

Eddie lost who he was, lost his spiritual core, as he gave away all that he had, hoping that others' praise would make him whole, esteemed, important. Because he had no center, the minute he faced what he saw as competition from his wife, he caved in on himself and came out frightened and fighting. Dealing from a less-than position, he did what he'd been taught to do: fight and break down what others had so that he wouldn't look so empty-handed. He shifted the focus from his own painful place of not being enough to his wife to a place where she wasn't enough herself. That's not balance; that's a zero-sum game in which zero tries to get the other person to be zero too.

Of course, that's not what it looked like to Eddie. In his eyes, he was giving her what she deserved for abandoning him, eclipsing him, and making him feel, in comparison, less like a man.

When you've lived an imbalanced life, everything you do is about deriving your worth, or regaining it, from what you do and not from who you are. It's about giving yourself away so completely that you hardly have a chance to develop a sense of self in the first place. Eddie has been giving away something that he shouldn't have parted with—himself—and the well has gone dry.

Lack of worth is the first cousin to inadequacy, but the two relatives are very different. Lack of worth tells you, "I'm not important; other people are far more important than I am." It says, "I prove my importance by showing others how important they are."

But taking care of other people and *not* taking care of yourself always come back to haunt you because if you've gone that route, like Eddie, you're fifty and looking at the prospect of no home and nothing to give to your children or grand-children. You remember all the stuff you've done for other people, but they've moved on now, and here you are with nothing but your rundown shoes and a beat-up car. You didn't take care of yourself, and all that hard work you did for others has left nothing to show for it. Sure, you have the inner joy and satisfaction of what you did, but while that has value, it doesn't overcome the reality of being fifty and having nothing to give to your grandchildren. Being fifty and feeling worthless.

So you're standing looking at yourself in the mirror and you say, "How do I know when I'm in this place of no self-worth?" When your feeling good is dependent on what you do for somebody else, you know you're in this place of no self-worth. And when you're resentful of people who do the same thing as you do and have gotten further along, you're in a place of no self-worth. You know you're in this place of no self-worth when you don't think you deserve material comfort for the work that you've done. When you've sold yourself for nothing, and you're angry about that.

It's not a comfortable place to be. Neither is it healthy. Anyone who lives in that place of no self-worth is prey to both fear and anger.

Transformation Plan and Power Tools

Eddie is a heartbreaker because this man is really a good man, a kind man. But he is now a deeply troubled, sad, and increasingly angry man. Because there is no core, the apple is rotting and starting to poison his relationships with himself, his wife, and his children.

The transformation here is complicated because basically what Eddie needs is an authentic, organic version of the self he has been all this time. But he needs real power and real worth for himself and for the world. He needs spiritual balance between who he is and what he does. Between his true being and his function in life. What he does has to flow from who he is as a person instead of just make up for his fear that he doesn't really amount to much that is worth anything.

Right now, Eddie feels like a victim. The initial power tools that he needs to transform his sense of having worked hard for nothing into a sense of spiritual purpose and power are the three A's: awareness, acknowledgment, and acceptance. Then he needs to add right action and stillness to his tool belt.

Awareness

Awareness is an internal process that relies on intuitive knowledge. It is the ability to identify and harness the spirit of truth. In Eddie's situation, that means he's going to have to have that inner sense that what he needs to do is build inner strength, inner worth, and inner direction that is separate and apart from what he does for other people. He's been giving other people worth and direction, but he hasn't given it to himself.

Awareness fosters consciousness of spiritual activity, and it opens mental and emotional faculties to the spirit of truth and to spiritual principles. It strengthens the faculty of belief, which is what Eddie needs right now—belief in himself.

In fact, the first thing he has to do is put himself first. This may seem selfish, but it isn't, because you can't give away what you don't have. If you put yourself first, you're more willing to take care of yourself. You won't need others to make up for what you can't give. The more you take care of yourself, the better you'll feel about yourself and everybody else. You've got to do what makes you feel good without depending on anybody else. You've got to be not selfish but self-ful. You've got to find a way—and for everybody that way will be different—to place yourself in the center without cutting everybody else out.

Acknowledgment

While awareness is a *process,* acknowledgment is more of an *action.* It's a demonstration of your willingness to accept truth as an active principle. Acknowledgment means owning what is yours. It eliminates human judgment and interpretation. It introduces the divine healing energy into life events. It strengthens a sense of freedom and independence. Acknowledgment is about recognition, and Eddie needs to recognize himself.

Acknowledge that your needs are as important as anyone else's. And see the imbalance in what's been going on. Whenever you're doing something for someone else, if you haven't done it for yourself, stop and do that first.

To do that, Eddie has to stop comparing himself to his wife. She is beside the point. All she has done is shine a spotlight on his sense of inner worthlessness and his lack of balance.

Don't compare yourself to others. Your insides and their outsides will never, ever match up. Don't compare where you are with where somebody else is. The moment you do that, you're going to feel less than the other person, and the comparison will raise static in your soul so that you won't be able to hear, think, or see clearly.

Instead of comparing, take an honest assessment of where you are in your life. Look at *your* side of the street, not theirs. Look at what you've done with your energy and your talent (and why you've done it). If Eddie looks at his life, he'll see that he's done great things for a great many people—for everyone, that is, except himself. He has to acknowledge that reality before he can move on.

Eddie has to do something that is only possible if he acknowledges that this is his problem, not someone else's. He has to embrace humility. It's not that you're not that powerful, but that you too are part of the world that needs to be saved. Since you can't give what you don't have, you can't give to your children because you don't have. So what are you really doing for the world? If he's denying himself, he's eventually not going to be able to give from a full cup. You've got to fill your cup and not depend on somebody else's misfortunes to be your fortunes.

Acceptance

The amazing thing about acceptance is that it's a psychological and emotional release of beliefs and thoughts. We all tell ourselves (and others) stories about who we are and what we do and why we do it, and our stories are just that: stories. "I did this for you because . . .", "I'm this way because . . .", "Such and such happened to me because ...", "I don't have this because ..." These aren't statements that have anything to do with reality; they're just stories we tell ourselves about a reality we imagine.

For Eddie, accepting reality is the key spiritual principle. If he can recognize both the power of truth—the *real* truth, not the truth he drafts for himself—and the presence of spiritual activity, he won't feel that he's a victim of a ball-busting wife, a worthless person who can't help his own kids, and a man in it all alone.

Acceptance facilitates transformation. It subdues the ego, which in Eddie's situation continually screams into his ear that everything is unfair and it's everyone else's fault that no one sees him and rewards him. If Eddie can accept that he himself set up his life to get some rewards that just aren't going to materialize, if he can accept the reality that this isn't about his wife, then that acceptance will create a shift in his attitude and in his consciousness.

Acceptance means finding a way to be okay with where you are, whoever you are. If you keep telling yourself stories in defiance of reality, you'll stay stuck in a one-down position for the rest of your life, and you'll be angry and resentful. If you can achieve acceptance, the anger and resentment will disappear.

Don't tell yourself stories!

Right Action

As simple as this sounds, a little right action will go a long way for Eddie. If he starts a college fund now for his grandkids, for example, and maybe takes out a small loan to help his son (paying it off regularly!), these things will help him move out of his all-or-nothing place. The way he sees things now, he's either all things to all people or he's dirt, the nothing of nothingness. A little right action, a little help here and there, will open Eddie's eyes to how many more choices he has than he thinks he has. The Quakers say, "When you pray, move your feet." Eddie has to do a little shuffling for an enormous reward: self-respect. Nothing creates balance faster than having a little substance inside.

Stillness

Stillness is the presence and activity of God within you and the willingness to surrender all that you are to that presence. It may seem like an odd tool for a man who feels that he isn't doing enough, but stillness is terribly important for Eddie because it will allow him into the presence of God.

Many of us experience stillness about four o'clock in the

morning, before the day gets busy. But we can (and should) bring ourselves into stillness at other times as well—into a state of quietness and oneness with the universe and with our own being.

How do we get to stillness in the chaos of today's world? Conscious breathing results in stillness, as does meditation (which is the art of stilling the mind). Learning how to *be* rather than what to *do* results in stillness of the ego, that part of us that breeds fear, doubt, anger, and the need to be in control. Living in the moment, casting off past regrets and fears for the future, results in stillness.

The reason Eddie needs stillness is that he needs to become bigger than his current situation, in which he feels smaller than everyone—particularly his wife. Eddie needs to know that he's enough in the moment, because only that will begin to restore balance. Tearing his wife down won't do it. That may provide a momentary relief, but regret will flood in after the anger recedes because deep down inside Eddie knows that this is *his* problem. Only in stillness and through quiet breathing can he become calm enough to hear that knowledge, to hear also that there's an answer to his problem of inadequacy. In calmness he can eliminate the human need to be in control and gain the sense of being whole. And that wholeness, that sense that he's enough, is the only thing that can balance him and his situation.

Seeking stillness may feel counterintuitive to Eddie—doing nothing to feel like something—especially since his wife is doing so much and he feels that he isn't doing enough. But it's *doing* that got Eddie into this jam in the first place. It's time to try a different way.

Knowledge Equals the Freedom to Choose

Eddie has to become self-assured, self-actualized, and self-reliant before he can be productive in any profession. A man can be a teacher, a cleric, a social worker, but if he's in a helping profession because he gets his sense of value and worth from helping other people, then he's destined for trouble. His motivation can't be compensatory.

Eddie has got to detach himself from the outcome of the people he helps. He's allowed himself to feel powerful through what others achieve with his support, but now, with his wife out-achieving him, he feels powerless again. The lack of balance in his life has been revealed by this reversal.

The good news for Eddie is that all people have been endowed with the ability to master themselves. You have this ability too. As we saw in the Introduction, it's a function of your connection to the Creator, to Spirit. The more you're aware, the more you acknowledge and accept your true identity, the more connected you'll be to Spirit. If you allow that connection to build, Spirit will show you that you can be complete in yourself if you stop, look, and surrender to your true nature.

Spiritual mastery, as I noted earlier, is a process of becoming conscious of and accountable for what you do under any given set of circumstances. It requires awareness of and adherence to spiritual principles as the motivating factors behind all your actions. This means controlling the responses of the human self and allowing natural laws and universal principles to stimulate your actions. Eddie's motivating factors are praise and recognition, not the spiritual principles that would make him whole. When he learns spiritual mastery, he'll be able to recognize when ego is at the helm and be able to put Spirit paramount again.

Stillness and conscious breathing help to subdue the ego and link the energy of the physical self with the energy of the spiritual self. That linking of energies works to create a balance between them. In the absence of balance, the ego reacts to any threat to its control by striking out (which often translates into putting your fist through the wall or screaming at your girlfriend). Because stillness and conscious breathing infuse the body with energy, they can subdue the ego and facilitate spiritual mastery over demanding urges whenever you slip out of balance.

It's human nature to respond to the ego's demands. As a human being, you're naturally motivated to listen to them. But spiritual mastery allows you to take control of any situation and subdue your conditioned response, to say to your anger, "Hey, wait! *I'm* in control here. You be still and quiet. I'm going to take care of you."

Contemporary culture wants you to believe that you're helpless and powerless to master the internal and external forces that affect your well-being. And certainly the ego-urge to tear someone down to build yourself up is strong, especially when it feels as if your very survival is at stake. But stop. Breathe. You don't need to say the destructive thing that first comes to mind; you don't need to do the destructive thing that first occurs to you. Good thing too, because destructive words and acts only make you feel smaller.

Eddie can stop his downward spiral. He can choose to become aware, to acknowledge what it is that's calling the shots inside him—that out-of-whack feeling, that sense of hollowness, that pervasive worthlessness. He can accept that that's what he's feeling and then be still, breathe in and out.

Take in his completeness in the eyes of the Divine and start some right action from that moment on.

There's an old saying that goes like this:

Begin where you are.
Do what you can gracefully do.
Step out in faith.
Expect God to help.

You don't have to do it all, and you don't have to do it alone.

Knowledge that you have the potential for spiritual mastery, that you can use the power tools discussed in this book to change how you live, gives you the freedom to make better choices. If you see yourself in Eddie, then stop right now. Choose your tools wisely from the array shown here and use them consistently.

If you have an Eddie in your life, don't do for him what he needs to do for himself. Don't buy the new car; don't buy the fancy clothes; don't pay for the gift to his kids. That sort of "help" just enhances his feeling that he can't provide what he wants and needs to provide. It doesn't support him in taking care of himself.

Unfortunately, our story of Eddie doesn't have a happy ending—at least not yet. Eddie is too stuck, at this point, to move from his competitiveness and anger. He can't drop his problem so that his hands are free to pick up the solution. He isn't willing to acknowledge why he so resents his wife for eclipsing him. His relationship, which would have been salvageable, is lost. He just can't accept divine help to make him balanced and whole.

It would be nice to tell you that Eddie did what Eddie had to do to change. And maybe I'll be able to say that someday. The solutions, the power tools of spiritual mastery, are just as available to him now as they ever were. Maybe losing his wife and *still* not being able to help his kids will make Eddie willing to work for improvement. I don't know. Only Spirit knows.

5

Gabriel

Not All Men Are Macho

How many fathers have tried to make their sons do a particular thing in a particular way because of what they thought they knew about the situation? How many mothers have warned their sons against behaving in a certain way because (as they like to point out) mothers can always see what's bound to happen? How many times have *you* acted or failed to act because you just *knew* what could happen? How many times have you given advice or attempted to stop or help someone because of what you feared would happen if the person continued along his or her path?

Well, Gabriel was stopped by his mother from being what he wanted to be because she just *knew* that no good could come of things she didn't see or hadn't experienced.

Instead of rebelling against his mother, Gabriel just goes with the flow. He's always been the kind of guy a girl calls "nice." He's not a standout guy, mind you—just an all-around regular guy who goes out of his way to be pleasant. He made it through high school and even college, but he wasn't a scholar and didn't play sports. Now he has a decent job in the accounting field, but he isn't raising any hell anyplace.

Gabriel had a few girlfriends during school and in his early twenties, but none of those relationships "stuck." He's been dating one woman off and on for the past eight years, but that relationship hasn't solidified either; in fact, both of them date other people fairly often.

Now, with an unnamed dissatisfaction rumbling through him, Gabriel is looking at himself critically and asking, "What am I doing here? Who am I?" Nice guy?

Now his mother is all over his case: "You're not good enough. You're not doing it right. Why aren't you married? Why don't you have children? You're in your mid-thirties already. Why can't you make a relationship work? And what's holding you up at work? Aren't you planning on moving up? You can't do *anything* right!"

That's certainly how it feels to him too, especially when it comes to women. His experience is that women want either more from him than he has or more than he's willing to offer. That's because he doesn't even register on the radar of *interesting* women—women who have something to offer *him*. Gabriel can't seem to figure out how to get the "edge" that he thinks the women he'd be interested in would want.

He has a brother who has that edge. Actually, it seems his brother has it *all*. His brother is married; he has the house, the car, the wife, the kids. He goes on vacation. In the Caribbean. The wife is a bit on the whiny side for Gabriel's taste—but his brother has got a relationship with this woman. He's not particularly fond of the way his brother treats her—they argue, they fight. He has affairs. But Gabriel is trying to just get *one* solid, steady relationship. He's a solid citizen, but he has to admit it, he's "nice." For crying out loud, he's even an accountant for a milk company! How NICE!

Gabriel feels he's not really making a statement with his life. The good thing about his job is he gets to meet women. He dates them and goes out. His crisis comes about because even though he's been dating women, he's been in one main relationship with a woman for eight years.

Although he's been involved with this woman for eight years, they've kept their lives pretty separate. And he's really enjoyed being able to go out with a lot of the women he's met through work. But now she's told him that unless he can commit to the relationship, she wants out. And he isn't sure what to do, because he's not sure how he feels about her.

And yet, does he love her? He's not really sure. For one thing, she has a tendency to overrun him. They almost always do what *she* wants to do; they go where *she* wants to go. And she's always pushing him: "Why do you stick with that job? Why don't you dress more savvy?" He feels rather henpecked by her, the same way he feels demoralized by his mother. So he finds that he's doing with his girlfriend what he does with his mother: always trying to prove that he loves her or to make her proud of him.

But now she wants to get married! After stewing about the issue for a few days, he finds that he isn't willing to marry her, because down deep inside of him, he doesn't feel that she's the best he can have; it's just that she's all he's *got*. No wonder it feels like a crisis!

Even though he's been proposed to, Gabriel still feels rejected. Somehow all of his "not good enough" buttons have been pushed. He feels as if he doesn't have anything to offer anyone. Head in hands, he asks himself, "What's wrong with me? I make a decent salary. I'm a decent person. I'm not blaz-

ing any new trails, but I'm not burning up any forests either."
His problem isn't so much with who he is to the outer world;
it's the inner work. He's not a mass-murderer and he's not a
company president or star athlete, but somehow he can't manage to be okay with just being okay.

Gabriel was a "good enough" man until he started looking
at his life. Now he floats between anger and depression. He
sits around the house puzzling over what to do about this
woman and her ultimatum.

The truth is, she's playing him like a fiddle. She's manipu-
lating him. She's trying to get him to do what she wants him to
do. He suspects that, but he's stuck anyway. He doesn't have
enough strength to say, "No, I won't do it that way," or enough
courage to say, "Yes, I will do it." She's running all over him,
and she'll keep doing it until he finds the courage and strength
to stick up for himself.

At some level he knows what she's doing, which makes the
issue a question of what *he* wants—and this is the problem.
Gabriel has always done what his *mother* wanted him to do.
That's how he got his identity, his approval, as he was matur-
ing, and now he doesn't know what he thinks about his own
life. The result is a depressed, powerless man who feels inadequate in his work and relationships.

Gabriel's problem is that he doesn't amount to much in his own eyes. When he looks at his older brother he sees a man who was able to send his wife to the Bahamas. Peter knows how to make a statement! He has other women on the side when he wants them, and he stands up to his wife when they disagree over things. He puts in his time running the Little League, but he can also go off to a boxing game with a bunch of buddies if he wants.

Gabriel doesn't have *any* of that. He has his job, which he likes well enough and from which he makes a decent salary. He has this woman, whom he likes well enough but isn't passionate about. But he doesn't have any savings; he has no house; he has no kids (and no money for them if he had them anyway!). He can take care of himself and his own little needs just fine. He certainly can't send his mama off on trips, though!

Talking to the Man in the Mirror

When Gabriel looks in the mirror, he sees a man in his mid-thirties who's got nothing to show for himself. He's done everything right, but just not right *enough*. He feels good, but not good *enough*. So he's at a crossroads: "Who am I? What's this about?"

If he wants things to change, he's going to have to take some action, whether he likes it or not. He's very passive typically, especially when he's doubting himself. "Maybe this is as good as it gets," he thinks, settling in to the status quo. But a part of him believes that he's entitled to better. He just doesn't know what to do to access it.

What's really going on with Gabriel is that he never found his true self. He did all the right things for all the wrong reasons. During his early life he wanted to be a veterinarian, but he didn't believe that he could make it through school. After all, his mother *told* him he couldn't. "Don't waste your time with more school," she said. "Get a job. You aren't the brains in the family." That was the job of his brother, of course, who went on to be a big-deal real estate salesman.

All Gabriel sees—all Gabriel has ever seen—when he looks at what defines success is Peter. He's out and about, meeting people. He's doing important things; he's in control; he has power. And his work gives him rewards. Peter is always talking about his commission on this deal or that. That's how he got to send his mother on her dream vacation. That's how he got his wife's sedan and his own car. In a world where the manliest men are also the men with the most money, in a world where power is measured in women and possessions, Gabriel is a mere shadow of his brother's man.

But Gabriel is starting to feel a bit defiant. He's realizing that he never stands up *in* himself *for* himself. He's so busy keeping his mother happy, holding down his job well, pleasing his girlfriend (even if he isn't sure she's the right one!), that he never does anything just for *him*.

Now he sees the rest of his life in front of him, and he thinks, "I don't like this. This isn't who I am. This isn't what I want." But the prospect of letting go of what he has brings up his fear of not knowing what's coming, and every time he thinks about an unknown future, he questions whether or not he can handle it.

The thing is, Gabriel hasn't really moved beyond the time when he was nineteen, a time when he was in a very oppressive relationship with his mom, by then a widow. His dad had been quiet, passive, for the most part, though Gabriel had sensed that he was full of an inner anger that he let out only in occasional bursts. Gabriel's father had had a heart attack and died when Gabriel was just barely a teen. After that, the young man felt as if he had to take care of his mother, do what she wanted, make her proud, fill his dad's shoes. Those shoes were really big, because his dad had provided for the family and taken care of them well, but the shoes pinched: his dad didn't have a voice. And neither does Gabriel. He's never found his voice, even in adulthood.

Gabriel's father's suppressed emotions took him to a heart attack. Gabriel is headed to the same place if he doesn't find the courage to stand up *in* his life *for* his life. He has to take those feelings of disillusionment and depression and put them at the center of his life for a moment, because they hold the energy, the fuel, to move him forward.

To live with these emotions, Gabriel needs self-acceptance. He needs courage. Trust is big for him too. Those who take the beaten path know where they'll end up, but those who make their own route don't always know. To break free of where he is, he needs to be able to ask things like, "Could I make it through veterinary school at this point in my life?"

My statement to him is, "Go find out!" At thirty-five, cut your mother's apron strings and go find out if you have the courage to deconstruct and then rebuild your life based on your ability to stand for what *you* want and who *you* are.

Gabriel doesn't have to prove to his mother that he loves her. Or that he's good enough. Or that he's his father. What he has to do is sit in the middle of all his depression and realize that he's being pushed down. That's what being *depressed* is!

What's weighing him down is his suppressed anger—anger that he barely knows he has. He's angry with his girlfriend for forcing the issue of marriage, and he's angry with himself for (a) not having the courage to stand up to his mother and his girlfriend, and (b) his ambivalence about his sibling. While he admires his brother, in another sense he despises him, because that model of manhood is not who he is. He's not the womanizing, outgoing power broker.

But what is the model for the gentler, softer, kinder man? What is that model? Not his father, certainly. Where do we find it? He didn't have one. Because the gentler, softer, kinder man who never spoke up to his demanding wife died of a heart attack. Now the gentler, softer, kinder Gabriel who didn't speak up to his demanding girlfriend is being left by this woman. He knows he's being manipulated by her, which makes him angry. He's angry at himself, he's angry at the world, he's angry at women, he's angry at men—he's just angry. But because he hasn't found his voice, he doesn't know how to appropriately express everything he's thinking and feeling. Disillusionment is the result: "I did everything right for the wrong reasons. I'm a decent guy, and nobody appreciates it."

Gabriel has to see he's powerless over these women. He tells himself, "They measure my worth by what I *do,* not by my *character*." And he'd be right. The truth that his *do* is not his *who* is lurking in the shadows, waiting for Gabriel to acquire the tools to discern it.

Transformation Plan and Power Tools

Gabriel is suffering from what he and society perceive as a certain lack of manliness. He isn't macho like Peter; he's softer and gentler. In our culture, softness connotes a lack of masculinity.

In the African tradition, males are taught from an early age the principles of manhood according to cultural prescriptions. The goal of the various rituals, ceremonies, and rites through which boys are taught to become men is to inspire, uplift, and support the development of consciousness. Young males are advised of their purpose in life, the things they were born to do. Not the specific things that society expects of them, but principles of the universal and natural laws that rule the flow of life and control the environment.

Armed with this information, males are then provided opportunities to demonstrate their ability to survive and support. They're also instructed in cultivating their God-given talents, gifts, and abilities at a pace that matches their temperament and is conducive to their purpose, and they're taught the importance of both the tangible and the intangible forces with which they'll interact in life.

This sort of manhood training is rarely available to males living in the Western Hemisphere today. If it were, Gabriel would have models and support for the kind of man he is: a nice guy, supportive and kind, totally lacking in macho instincts. He would feel comfortable with who he is.

What can Gabriel do to improve his fit in the world, to make himself more comfortable? In a society where a successful male looks more like his brother than like Gabriel, does he have to transform who he is to become adequate? No. Transformation is needed, yes, but what must be transformed is how Gabriel feels about himself. He has to get from a place where others judge him to be insufficient to a place where he knows he's exactly who Spirit meant him to be. His task—the task of *all* men, really—is to divine his gifts and his purpose so that he can feel complete in himself just as he is.

And there's help for Gabriel. The spiritual power tools— especially awareness, acknowledgment, and understanding— will help him change his outlook and his self-image.

Awareness

Gabriel's first power tool, awareness, involves serious self-reflection. In workshops I give, I engage participants in a mirror exercise. I ask them to establish eye contact with themselves in a mirror and assess what they see. Almost without fail, participants smooth their eyebrows, fix their hair, or closely scan their face for pimples. Those who are able to establish the eye contact—and not all are!—have one of two reactions: they look away quickly, or they cry.

We haven't been taught how to take the time to look at ourselves, to be with ourselves. We're conditioned to *polish the shell,* to make ourselves look good for the world. When we see (or, more important, *feel*) the energy of who and what we are, we're humbled. "The eyes are the mirror of the soul," says an ancient adage. The eyes are also the principal connection to the mind. Thus the first step toward personal empowerment is the ability to connect with and see yourself. This ultimately results in acknowledgment of who you are and begins the development of the spiritual mind.

For Gabriel to turn his life around, he first has to look deeply at himself in that mirror; he has to look without flinching and find the place where he gave himself away. Was it at age nineteen, when he went toward business as opposed to pre-med? Was it even earlier, when he took his mother's daughter's friend to the prom instead of the girl he wanted to take? Or both these times, and others too? Where exactly did he lose himself?

Once Gabriel has made that determination, he's got to allow himself to go back to the past, look at his choices, and make peace with them. Then he's got to reinvest himself in his own dream.

Acknowledgment

Acknowledgment is key to Gabriel's transformation. Gabriel has to acknowledge his feelings, his sense of not being "good enough." He's got to acknowledge the compromises he's made that have dishonored him. He's got to acknowledge the times in his relationship with his mother and with the other women in his life when he hasn't stood up *in* himself *for* himself.

Furthermore, he's got to acknowledge the payoff: what he got for giving himself up was that he didn't have to take risks. He didn't have to risk disappointing or upsetting people—notably, his mother. Rather than risk upsetting anyone, he was willing to lose himself. He swallowed his voice and cut himself off from his true self. He stopped being seen for who he was and became visible only by his compliance.

In fact, his compliance is so prominent that it completely hides his anger—an anger that still festers because Gabriel feels trapped by his circumstances, controlled by others, and helpless to change the course of his life. Now he needs to acknowledge the anger and work to direct it appropriately.

Gabriel is trapped by concerns of the ego—concerns such as anger—and that's a problem, because the ego and human will (which develop in response to experiences and judgments about experiences) aren't in line with universal law. Will and ego are centered on the way things "appear" to be, which is only a portion of what things really are. They create conflict in the mind, which then feeds into the emotional being as fear, anger, depression, and other goodies such as envy, hate, and greed.

Acknowledging all the forces at war inside him will give Gabriel the energy to move forward instead of feeling beaten down by things he doesn't want to look at, acknowledge, or accept.

Understanding

Gabriel has got to really understand himself. That's the only way he'll be able to separate out what he does or doesn't do from who he truly is, from his essential nature. He may have to ask himself probing questions repeatedly—ten or fifteen or a hundred times—before he begins to shape his answers. And he must do all this without comparing who he is to anybody else.

He'll want to ask himself all of the following, and more: Who am I? What is it that makes me tick? What kinds of things make me feel bad about myself? What kinds of things make me feel good about myself? How have I compromised those feel-good things? Why did I do it? What was I going for? Did I get the payoff I was hoping for? And when I got it, was it what I wanted?

Remember that big friend of mine who was so afraid of the bee that he lost sight of the fact that he was hitting me with a three-pound book? If he'd understood the power of his fear, he would have understood that the harm he was inflicting on me was far worse than any damage the bee could have done. And like my friend, Gabriel is hitting himself over the head because he doesn't understand the forces that are paralyzing and depressing him.

Gabriel has to now understand, really *understand,* that he's been running away from risk and that he pays a heavy price for that in his soul. Once he achieves that understanding, he's got to decide whether he's willing to keep paying that price or whether he'd rather learn to deal with risk. There's always been an advocate within him saying things like, "Let her go! She's not the woman for you." Or "Make your own decisions. *Let* your mother be upset." Or "*Let* your brother call you a wuss." Perhaps it's time now to listen to that voice within.

Gabriel once had a clear vision of where he wanted to go: veterinary medicine. What might his voice within say to that vision now? "Call for a program catalog today. See how long the coursework would take. Or if you can't go to vet school, could you be a veterinary assistant? Could you work for the SPCA? Could you be a dog-walker? Or is it maybe time to let that dream go and find a new one?"

Let me offer an aside to all you women out there who've ended up with these kinder, gentler men. We women need to understand that we have to create and support broader models of masculinity, so that we're reasonable in what it is that we demand and expect of the men in our lives. Comparing them all to weight lifters and boxers, as we do now (metaphorically anyway), doesn't make them better men, just men who feel less valuable than others. We need to value our men for who they are, not for what they do. And we need to be mindful of our tendency to make men prove themselves to us. This is especially key for mothers, who must allow sons to be sons, not try to fit sons into a mold they (or their spouse) create.

Knowledge Equals the Freedom to Choose

At all times in this life, two plans are operating. The first is the plan of the human mind, which teaches us that only the strong survive, only the smart make it. The human plan says that you compete for your place in life, though you're not given all the rules for the competition. The human plan is that you live hard and grab all you can get. If you're among the lucky few, the human plan gets you to where Gabriel's brother got: outward success.

The other plan is the plan of Spirit. It is Spirit's plan that you see that all people have a well-ordered life and live abundantly. It is a plan designed to teach you that although lessons and tests will occur in life, there's a wellspring of knowledge within your being; an unlimited source of inspiration, protection, and guidance is always available to you. In that spiritual plan, the blueprint for choosing is there, at your fingertips.

Understanding will give insight. Insight will help Gabriel see that emotions undiagnosed and out of control cause disaster. Emotions understood and harnessed cause freedom and power.

The plan of Spirit is the plan that Gabriel has to turn to now. He swallowed who he was in following the human plan of his mother; now, with the help of Spirit, he can make better choices in accordance with the spiritual plan.

With the help of the spiritual power tools, he'll be able to understand and harness his emotions, gaining freedom and power. He'll be able to turn his fear of being nothing into the strength to become something very special indeed, and he'll be able to turn his anger into energy.

This society doesn't value the kind, gentle man as overtly as it does the alpha macho man. Gabriel, to survive and to implement Spirit's plan for him, will need to value himself. If he can learn to see his situation as valuelessness in his mother's or girlfriend's eyes as opposed to real worthlessness, if he can learn to see that he doesn't fit into the macho mold but nonetheless has inherent worth, he'll find the courage and the strength to please himself first and then worry about the rest of the people in his life.

Once he's learned to see the value in himself, he'll go out and associate with people who value that best self. He'll find things to do that are of value to him, even if they don't look very masculine.

After many long months of pain and despair, Gabriel finally saw what he had to do. He let his girlfriend go (though he was nice to the end), and he cut off communication with his mother until he could find a way to be in relationship with her that honors himself. Instead of calling her almost daily, he started sending her cards every so often. He changed his phone number and didn't give the new one to her because he wanted to stop her constant badgering.

What these actions show is that he decided to opt for risk over safety. For example, he took the risk of upsetting his mom so that he could begin to feel okay in himself. That was very hard for him—a classic middle-of-the-road guy.

He started looking at veterinary schools, but he also pursued options tied to his accounting work. He was promoted to head of his accounting department not long after the transformation process began. While he was deciding what he wanted to do in the long term, he started doing little things that spoke to his deepest desires. He started an animal-petting program for children with AIDS, for example.

Once Gabriel saw his situation clearly, once he accepted his part in it, he came unstuck from his mother's vision of his life. He began evaluating for himself what he did and didn't want, and for the first time since his late teens he was able to feel that what he had to contribute was as worthy and as "manly" as anyone else's contribution.

6

Martin

Taking Care of Unfinished Business

It wouldn't be accurate to say that Martin simply walked out on his wife of eight years and their two sons, aged five and three. It would be more accurate to say he left in stages.

The first stage was entertaining the idea. Martin had come to the point where he realized that he simply didn't want to be married anymore. The truth is, he couldn't stand up to the pressure of being responsible (and *feeling* responsible) for three other lives. More important, he couldn't stand the feeling that he wasn't adequately living up to his responsibilities as a husband and father. His wife's constant nagging and complaining about what he ought to or shouldn't do and what he needed to do more or less didn't help the situation.

The second stage was exploring the possibility (and the experience) of actually being gone. For Martin, that meant having somewhere else to go. Enter the girlfriend. She made it easy for Martin to stay away from home in stages. First one night, then a weekend, then longer. Depending on how angry (or sad) his wife was when he went back home, Martin would up (or lower) the ante. If his wife screamed and issued ultimatums when Martin returned from one of his getaways, he used her behavior as an excuse to storm out and stay gone for weeks; if she cried, he would lie, make love to her, and stay home for a week or two, using the kids as an excuse to get away from his girlfriend. (She knew he was married; she just didn't know *how* married.)

He'd call every now and then just to check in when he was away, but he'd hang up if his wife started in on him again. Her anger gave him a reason to stay away. Her tears had the opposite effect: if she cried, the tears always brought him home. He rarely allowed himself to think about his sons, because that made the pain unbearable. He knew that his wife would tell them *something* to explain his absences, and whatever the explanation was, he'd deal with its ramifications later.

The third stage was to actually leave—to go home, gather the things that mattered most to him, and walk away. Martin had had some practice with this stage, because he'd helped his brother Joe leave *his* family. Joe had made his getaway on a Sunday morning. Martin had sat in the car as his brother packed and walked boldly out the door, slamming it behind him. He'd been able to hear his sister-in-law and the children screaming and then sobbing in the background. Martin remembered that his brother had cried too, just like a baby, once he'd gotten in the car. He also remembered that by the time he'd dropped his brother off at *his* girlfriend's house, his sister-in-law had been put in her place; in his brother's mind, she was a nagging, conniving bitch who'd tried to suck him dry and had never been satisfied.

Many of Martin's friends had had similar experiences. They simply couldn't satisfy their wife's demands, and both the demands and the failure to measure up made them angry. It didn't matter that many of the things the women pointed out were true; what mattered was that they were always pointing it out. The nagging, whining, and complaining made Martin's friends feel inadequate. No man likes to be beat over the head with his shortcomings.

No man likes name-calling either, but in Martin's experience, wives seem to love it. They fling out labels such as *irresponsible, insecure,* and *immature*—labels all but guaranteed to ensure that a man doesn't feel good about himself. So what if the wife's assessment is, in many cases, true? Who wants to be called irresponsible and then be expected to turn over his paycheck?

Like Martin, many of his friends had realized that girlfriends rarely complain during the first year. It usually takes them a while to start making demands. If a guy plays his cards right, he can get himself together and be ready to move on before the demands begin. Where and how he moves is of less importance than *that* he moves. Martin was counting on his girlfriend to be true to form. He needed to work out a plan, but that would take time. Because in his experience girlfriends are more willing than wives to give a guy the time he needs, he figured that he had to leave home for good and settle in with his girlfriend.

Martin didn't feel as brave as his brother or some of his friends, who'd taken the direct approach with their wives. Instead, praying that his wife hadn't changed the locks, he decided to make his escape when she wasn't there. He picked a time when he knew she'd be at work (and the kids at daycare) and skulked up to the house. Recognizing that there would be major fallout from his actions, he was almost sorry when the key turned in the door.

Stepping inside, he felt a wave of regret over what he was giving up, but he swallowed it and set to work. He gathered his favorite clothes and a few other things that he really needed. He took a picture or two for their sentimental value. Other than that, he left his wife everything. After all, that seemed to be what she wanted: she wanted things, not a man. She wanted a servant who would respond to her every beck and call. She wanted much more than Martin had, more than he was willing to give.

Martin had tried at first to be all that his wife wanted; he really had. But when he'd failed, she'd beat him up about it. He knew that *she* knew that he had another woman. Yet instead of trying to make him feel better so that he'd come back to her, she chewed him out and threatened him. Didn't she know that it was all her fault? Didn't she know that it was her lack of appreciation, her lack of support, her constant nagging and complaining that had driven him out of her bed? Didn't she know that he was doing his best—had been for most of a decade!—and it was never enough? After eight years, didn't she know what he needed and how to give it to him?

Martin concluded—as he'd concluded so many times in the recent past—that she didn't, and that he had a right to leave since it was his wife's fault that he felt inadequate. But that conviction didn't make the process easy. Like his brother, Martin cried as he left the house. First he cried aloud, mourning the loss of family; then later, and often, he cried to himself. Eventually, though, he put his wife in her place mentally. As for his kids, he decided he'd deal with the fallout with them later; he wasn't up to seeing them just yet.

In the months that followed his departure, Martin dealt with dozens of harassing calls from his wife. Sometimes she called to chew him out, and they'd both end up mad. Other times, though, she'd call in a moment of weakness and tearfully beg him to come home. On those occasions, he'd always promise to stop by to see the kids, though he rarely kept those promises.

A few times his wife showed up at his girlfriend's house. When that happened, Martin let the two women fight it out. It was easy to sidetrack his wife from his own behavior when she was busy blaming the girlfriend, so he never tried too hard to make them get along.

Eventually the calls and visits stopped, and Martin was both relieved and frightened. Because his wife wasn't nagging him anymore, he started sending checks to help with household expenses. When she called to tell him that he wasn't sending *enough* money, he cut her off again.

It took his wife years to divorce him. By that time, Martin

had been through four girlfriends, leaving each one in stages once the demands and name-calling began. When he finally did settle down and remarry quite a few years later, his sons were already fifteen and seventeen. His ex-wife and her boyfriend had been together for eight years by then. Although they'd never gotten married, the man had raised Martin's sons. It didn't make Martin feel good, but he had to respect the guy for what he'd done.

Martin had a new family now. Two daughters and another son. His second set of children knew nothing about the first set. He had decided that they did not need to know. He and his second wife owned a home. Although Martin had a girlfriend here and there, he and his wife were doing pretty well.

Then one day Martin received the telephone call that he'd been dreading for most of his adult life. His oldest son called, wanting to see him because his younger brother was in trouble. Martin didn't ask for any details; he didn't think he had a *right* to ask. Besides, his son had made it very clear that he wanted to know only one thing: Why? Why had he left them? Why hadn't he kept his promises? Why hadn't he ever sent so much as a *birthday* card? His son added that *he* didn't care, but his brother needed to know. He went on to explain that the younger son had tried twice to commit suicide. The older boy thought that it was because of his anguish over Martin's abandonment, so he came to Martin to get the whys.

Now Martin was really in a fix. The thing he'd been running from for years—taking responsibility for his actions, his feelings, *everything*—was staring him dead in the face.

Talking to the Man in the Mirror

The lesson in all of this is that we're held accountable for what we do. We can avoid accountability for a while, but sooner or later whatever we run away from will catch up to us. Like Martin, if we run away from our past and our responsibilities, we'll lose our identity and be left with only that vague phantom-limb feeling that comes from hacking half one's life off.

Martin started running away emotionally long before he actually did it physically, as we saw earlier. His wife's complaints projected his own unspoken fears about himself. When he heard his wife talk about his inadequacy, her comments reinforced his own fear—the fear that he was inadequate. That's the key here: that feeling of inadequacy. While it looked to Martin as if all of his troubles came from the outside, they really came from inside—from that selfsame feeling of inadequacy.

And how did he respond to that feeling? He blamed. Not

himself, of course; he blamed his wife for telling him over and over again that he wasn't good enough, didn't give enough emotionally, physically, or financially. He blamed the kids too; he blamed the girlfriends; in fact, he blamed everyone *but* his own self. The blame got so big and so loud that in his view it justified his running away from everyone.

Now, facing a potential crisis with his sons, he's hearing his own inner thoughts come back to him in his ex-wife's voice. All he can hear is her rebuke for all the years he was absent. In her absence, he's telling himself, "I'm not doing enough. I'm not being enough. *I'm not enough.*" Her words of years ago are now his, and he's mirroring them back to himself.

One day he decides to call her to see what she knows about the kids' concerns. When he finally reaches her, she claims—no surprise—that it's his fault because he didn't do enough. But even if *she* hadn't accused him, *he* would have. He's living proof that you can run for years, but your life will mirror back to you your own inner talk wherever you go.

As Martin looks at himself in the mirror and takes stock, he hasn't a clue what's really going on. After all, he's built up a years-long argument that it's all *her* fault. He *can* see, though, that he's in trouble and has to change, because what he sees is this:

For all his fleeing and searching, he still isn't satisfied with himself or his life.

He can't look his sons in the face, though he yearns to be someone they can look up to.

He can't look his ex-wife in the face, though there was a time that face could bring a smile to his own without even trying.

As Martin thinks about these issues, it dawns on him that he never stuck up for himself with his ex-wife when they were married. He never pointed out what he *was* doing when she pointed out what he *wasn't*. He was content to let her beat up on him, as long as he could then make her out to be a complete bitch. That way she was in the wrong and he didn't have to take responsibility for himself.

Martin's passivity has led to something else besides blame: tremendous self-doubt and corrosive guilt. He walked out of that first marriage without finding or making the courage to face his demanding ex-wife. He deliberately walled himself off from her and from the kids, but as a consequence he gave up any chance of personal redemption. He sealed his failure by never going back and trying to do the right thing.

Both Martin and his first wife missed the opportunity to work through and learn from their mistakes. The problems that escalated into a divorce weren't all on *either* side of the street. (They rarely are.) Both partners shared in what brought them together in love, and both shared in what brought them down. While Martin may indeed have shown irresponsibility at times, his wife never learned to express her feelings and ideas without criticism. And neither one of them bothered to affirm the love between them.

Now that Martin faces a point of crisis, he has another chance to learn from his mistakes. With the help of the spiritual power tools, he can begin to rebuild the relationships that he was so instrumental in destroying.

Transformation Plan and Power Tools

The moral of this story is that what you do comes back to bless or haunt you, so you've got to be clear about what you're doing. If you're blaming other people and outside circumstances, if you're not taking responsibility, and if you're not honoring yourself and others, eventually those acts are going to come back to you. A lot of men discover this, but few know how to deal with it. Like Martin, they feel for years the guilt and shame and fear of their unfinished business.

Martin is one of the lucky ones. He gets the opportunity to transform his guilt into freedom because his son's return bearing grim news pierces Martin's protective coating of blame just long enough that he can see past his ex-wife's bad behavior to his own part. Once the blame drops away, the shame floats up. To be transformed, Martin now has to take those feelings of shame and guilt and build a life around taking responsibility.

Martin's spiritual crisis is his chance to right a serious wrong. It's his chance to show that he understands the spiritual law of the universe: we're held accountable for what we do. His primary tools in the transformation ahead are awareness, acknowledgment, confession, surrender, forgiveness, and responsibility.

Awareness

Avoiding guilt, shame, and blame, Martin has to strive to become aware so that he can make more enlightened and productive choices. He has—and has always had—the ability and the right to choose what he thinks and how he responds. Awareness enhances that ability and enlarges the scope of that right.

As long as we're thinking about, ducking under, and dodging the unpleasant physical experiences that we perceive to be lurking around every corner, we're powerless. Our real power lies within the self—lies in Spirit as it dwells within our being—which always has our best interests and protection in mind. Martin has to trust that awareness will bring him power.

Acknowledgment

Martin must do the one thing that he's resisted mightily over the years: face his fears, face his life, face his feelings of inadequacy. As long as Martin has blamed his ex-wife—fairly or unfairly—he's been able to sweep under the rug his feelings of not having been a father to his sons. He's discovered, though, what we noted earlier: that if you fail to acknowledge inappropriate behaviors, they become anchors around your neck. They weigh you down and hold you back. They make you angry at all the people you blame for what you've done. They put you in the role of victim, and in that role you give away your power.

Once you acknowledge to yourself what you've done, how you have or haven't responded, you become aware of specific behaviors that aren't productive. And once you acknowledge that those behaviors aren't working, you're once more in a position to make choices in your life, and you open yourself up to healing.

Because Martin didn't acknowledge his responsibility to his sons for so many years, the wounds in him have festered, infecting him with pain and poison and corrosive inadequacy. Opening up those wounds may hurt a bit at first, but even the foulest sores can be cleaned out and healed. By acknowledging that he's been hiding, that he's been irresponsible, Martin opens himself up to healing.

Confession

Martin must not only acknowledge his feelings to himself, lest they crash in on him. He must also tell his *sons* the absolute, unabashed, radical truth and be willing to deal with the fall-out. If he tells one lie here, at this crucial juncture, his world is going to crumble. He can't cover up a lie with another lie; it just doesn't work.

Remember that there are two really powerful results of confession: first, it frees the mind of guilt; second (in the absence of guilt), it disarms your defense mechanisms. When you have no guilt, your self-esteem rises and you don't feel compelled to defend yourself. When you don't need to defend yourself, you don't need to get angry or blame others.

For Martin there's an additional positive outcome of confession: if he confesses his shortcomings and failings, then his ex-wife and sons can't use them against him. The accusations will lose their power.

Surrender

Instinctively, Martin knows that surrender is important. Because he can't alter facts, he's wasting valuable energy every second that he fights them. One son is in deep trouble and the other is raging mad. Those are givens, as are the years of history between the father and sons.

For Martin, surrender takes a tremendous act of courage and power, but it's a turning point toward healing. It creates a shift in his consciousness from powerless human being to child of Spirit, entitled to all the help in the universe.

Forgiveness

At the time Martin left home, he was doing the best he could. He had a choice back then: face the fear and tell the truth, or don't face it and run away. He wasn't ready; he simply wasn't. But like all of us, he eventually had to face what he ran from. A fight like that requires spiritual stamina, along with the ability to embrace and practice truth, humility, and honor. But those spiritual principles are mere pie-in-the-sky theories until we're able to admit that we did our best and forgive ourselves where we fell short.

By forgiving, we clear our mental and emotional airwaves so that we can move on and do better. Martin has to forgive his ex-wife and himself before anything else can happen. This is the hardest part of the healing process for him, because he knows that he really did wrong by his sons. Each time he gets stuck on forgiveness—and it happens a lot—he has to go back and surrender some more to the fact that he did what he did and it can't be undone.

Spirit is all-knowing and all-forgiving. The more Martin moves toward creation of his own spiritual identity, the more readily and fully he'll be able to forgive.

Responsibility

Remember that responsibility is synonymous with power. Taking responsibility is the only way to have power psychologically, emotionally, and spiritually. If Martin takes responsibility for everything that's going on in his life, he'll have the power to make the changes that are needed.

The responsibility-power relationship is especially important in Martin's case, because his feeling of inadequacy is so strong. Somehow he has to challenge his feeling of not being up to the task of fatherhood and believe that he's adequate. There's only one way to do that successfully, and that's by taking responsibility.

Martin needs to take responsibility not only for what he did in the past but for his present actions. If Martin tells a lie to his sons now, he'll create *another* difficult experience that eventually will have to be dealt with. But the minute he admits to his part in everything, he'll regain the ability to choose how he feels and responds. When responsibility is taken, power floods in.

Knowledge Equals the Freedom to Choose

When a lie—or a series of hundreds upon hundreds of lies—comes back to you, you've got to take the higher ground. You've got to be willing to face somebody's anger. You've got to be willing to face your own shame. You've got to be willing to face your own guilt. Martin thought of calling his ex-wife to ask her what she had told her sons all these years. He realized it didn't matter. Nothing she could say would help him through this. The "later" had finally caught up with him. The courage he couldn't find back then, he would have to find now. On his way to work on the day of the meeting, Martin put his head on the steering wheel and cried like a baby.

He knew that defensiveness wouldn't work. Neither would blaming or lying. Those had failed him before. He couldn't put the agony of the breakup on anybody but himself. He had to take full responsibility for his actions. He had to tell the truth, because the truth would set him free. There was risk, to be sure: it was possible that after this meeting he'd have no relationship with his sons. The one committing suicide is going to bring up all the feelings of guilt and shame. So where he was blaming his wife before, he has to be very careful not to blame himself now, but to actually tell the truth.

The question for Martin is, When the lie comes back in your face some years down the road, how are you going to handle it *this* time? What choices are you going to make *this* time? What are you ready and willing to do *this* time?

If Martin looks honestly at his life, he'll see that he's already dispelled the myth that he's inadequate, because he has another wife, another set of kids, and a relationship that's working. So all the stuff that he thought he couldn't do—that his first wife's critical approach *convinced* him he couldn't do—he's proven he *can* do.

The fact of the matter is, the inner question is, How do you not dishonor yourself? And how do you confront your own feelings of inadequacy, shame, and guilt without blaming anybody else?

Using the power tools, Martin was able to confess his part in the dissolution of his family without placing blame on either himself or his wife. His older son listened but was too angry to accept Martin's offer to help in any way he could. Martin then arranged to see the younger son as well. They had a strained meeting, but Martin walked away from it knowing that he'd done the right thing at last. The conversations may or may not have helped either son, but they were a blessing to Martin: he became aware of a lightness within him, a beginning of peace in a deep place, and a sense of being connected to the all-healing, all-knowing power that comes only when we see our true connection to Spirit.

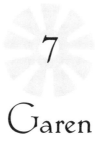

7

Garen

What Makes a Man

Standing there, looking at her, his heart melted. She was exquisite. As Garen watched her sleeping, his mind raced, flooded with thoughts of their future together and of the love that would grow between them. It was nothing short of awesome! Feeling a bit misty-eyed, he looked around to make sure that no one was watching him watch her.

Realizing that he was being watched, his heart went cold. His thoughts flipped from love to disgust and disdain. Shoving his hands into his pockets, he shifted his gaze out the window. In the same moment, from somewhere in the pit of his stomach, came the sour taste of shame; guilt and anger slithered their way into his brain matter. The loving, peaceful, silent exchange he had been having with his new love was now gone. In its place, stomping through his brain like a four-year-old having a temper tantrum, was a single thought: *Damn! How did I get myself into this? Again?*

As beautiful as she was, his four-day-old daughter represented his uncanny ability to put himself into a situation he knew he had no business being in. A situation that he'd promised himself he *would not* put himself in. But here he was again. Staring at another one of his children—the third one—trying to figure out how he could have the child in his life without letting yet another mother run his life.

Unfortunately, the child's mom had other ideas. There she was, staring at him. Talking to him. Trying to convince him that things would be fine if he'd just do what she was asking him to do.

Why is she even talking to me? he thought. *Doesn't she realize that I've just had a baby? Doesn't she realize that I feel weak and vulnerable right now—extremely vulnerable? Why is she stressing me now?*

"Who do you think she looks like?" the baby's mother asked.

"Well, she doesn't look anything like *me,* that's for sure!" he shot back.

"What the hell is *that* supposed to mean?" Mama Bear had her fur in a dander now.

"It means whatever you think it means!" He moved away from the bed so that the yelling wouldn't wake the sleeping angel. He knew that he was about to make his exit. He also knew that it wouldn't be pretty.

"Are you saying that she isn't yours?" Her voice was harsh with anger and shock. "Are standing there telling me that you don't believe you're this baby's father?" She was screaming now.

Unwilling to commit fully one way or the other, he responded by saying, "You brought it up. I didn't."

Damn, he hated this part! He hated having to resort to demonstrating his disregard for the women he slept with. He hated watching them cry. He hated them for making him resort to such measures. More important, he hated himself for putting himself in a position where he was forced to act this way.

"Look, you called me, and I'm here," he said. "You asked me to come see your baby, and I came. I told you before that it doesn't make sense to me that you'd have a baby with a man you hardly know. I have no way of knowing if this kid is mine or not. If you say it is, I guess I have to believe you, but that doesn't mean I have to accept you or the child."

She was crying now. "You know, you're a real piece of . . ."

"Watch your mouth! I told you before that you don't have the right to talk to me any old way you choose. And please stop calling my house. My girlfriend doesn't like it. I'm not bothering you, so why do you keep bothering me?"

Knowing that this was where it was going to get really hard, he started moving toward the door.

"How *can* you?" she said, sounding deflated. "How can you talk to me like this? How can you deny your child like this?"

It wasn't easy, but he'd had some practice. "I'm not denying anything," he said. "I'm simply saying I don't know for sure that she's mine, and you refuse to prove anything."

Knowing that he'd destroyed her pride and her fantasy, he moved in for the kill. "I'll tell you what. If you decide that you don't have anything to hide and you want me to take a blood test, give me a call. Call me at work, though. I'll see what I can do to help you out. If she's mine, I'll do what I'm supposed to do for her. Let me know—and take care of yourself."

On the other side of the door, he stopped for a moment to let the nausea in his gut subside. Walking down the stairs, he tried to recapture the sight of her face—not the mother's face, the baby's face. It was *his* face. It was the face of his two other children. Realizing that he just wasn't ready to stay, to try, to commit, or to fail, he allowed the face to fade from his brain.

It would be okay. *This* mother was too proud to cause trouble. She wasn't like his son's mother, who constantly hounded him and badgered him. His son's mother had taken him to court. This one wasn't like that one. This one would never even call now, after that last conversation; he'd put money on it. She'd raise his child alone, or perhaps with another man, but she wouldn't ask *him* for help. It didn't matter. Well, it *did,* but it didn't, because he *knew* that he couldn't handle the responsibility or the guilt or the truth.

He might mess up the way his father had messed up. He might get hurt the way his father had gotten hurt. He sometimes wondered if he could be a father, a decent one, but he knew that he'd likely be hurt, and he couldn't stand the thought of that.

As he drove away, leaving his daughter behind, he promised himself that he'd never sleep with another woman without protection. It was the same promise he'd made to himself on many, many occasions in the past. This time, though, he really believed that he meant it.

Talking to the Man in the Mirror

Fear is like a growling dog that has you pinned to a wall. When you move, it growls louder. Holding yourself as still as if paralyzed, you watch the little droplets of saliva as they fall from the dog's mouth. Though you try to empty your mind of thought, you imagine what will happen to you if you move again. You visualize the dog ripping at various parts of your body. You can actually feel the pain of the dog's teeth tearing through your flesh. With your eyes locked on the dog's gaze, you try to convince yourself that you'll get away, that you *can* get away, knowing that if you so much as sneeze, the four-legged beast is going to rip you apart.

When something happens in your life, how you respond is based on your perception of your ability to handle that particular situation. All that you've observed, experienced, and been taught, and the faith you place in your abilities, either supports or conflicts with your perceptions.

Abilities grow, become enhanced through practice. That's the natural course of things. However, if you get stuck in the perception of a particular ability, that ability isn't able to grow. It will atrophy, and you'll become stagnant.

Whenever you're faced with a situation that calls for a response, you must practice your ability to negotiate your way through whatever it is that's going on. You must navigate through your mental and emotional realities in order to make your way through the physical reality.

When you add fear to the equation, your ability to respond—your *response-ability*—is lessened. In fact, under extreme circumstances it's totally diminished. That's why whenever what you tell yourself about your ability convinces you that there's an increased possibility of pain, failure, or some other form of mental or emotional discomfort, fear rather than choice becomes the ruler.

When fear is present in your consciousness, you're reluctant to examine your choices, believing that you'll be called on or forced to do something you're afraid to do. So what do you do? You *react* rather than *respond*—and your reaction is nothing more than avoidance of the perceived pain or danger.

Of course, the pain or danger you perceive may be very real indeed. There really may be a growling hound dog standing in front of you, as real as the nose on your face. The issue is, *Does the dog have teeth? Can the dog outrun you? Can you call out to the owner? Is the place you're in the place you're supposed to be in, or are you out of place? Is that why the dog has confronted you?*

When you're afraid, these questions may not occur to you. If you have no faith in your ability to respond to a particular danger, they're irrelevant to you; you *know* that you're done for. But if you have faith in your ability to respond, these are exactly the sort of questions you'll ask.

The only way out of fear is through it. That's right! You have to test the dog. You have to make a run for it! You have to take a chance on being bitten or even mauled. Yes, it could be painful, but look at the alternatives. How long are you going to stay smashed to the wall? And what if you stay absolutely still but the dog bites you anyway?

Is it getting bitten that you're really afraid of? Or are you afraid that you won't be able to *handle* getting bitten? I'd suggest that for most of us, it's the latter. We place no faith in our ability to handle a situation because we use all of our strength trying to avoid or deny that the situation even exists. When something comes up, we react rather than respond, because we haven't developed and practiced our abilities enough to have confidence that we'll know exactly what to do.

We put our faith in what we've seen others attempt to do. We put our faith in our own failed attempts and the attempts of others. We rely on what happened the last time, or what could happen.

Fear tells us that whatever could happen that is bad and painful will surely happen. The problem is that we believe it will happen, and we govern ourselves accordingly. As related to the male psyche, the challenge is intensified because the male mind always relies on logic. It seeks a rational approach to the present situation. It may seem completely irrational to kick the dog and run for your life. Then again, most men would never admit that they run away in fear, because that is completely irrational!

How can a man abandon his child? When the fear is great enough, he can do just what Garen did: lie through the teeth and avoid responsibility.

How can so many men father children and walk away? How can they relinquish responsibility for the children they've co-created? I've spoken to hundreds of men about this issue. Many of them offered lame excuses, and most expressed a great deal of blame and anger. "I didn't want to have a baby!" "She just had that baby to trap me!" "She told me she was on the pill!" "I can barely take care of myself, let alone a kid." "She had the baby. I told her to have an abortion. It's her responsibility."

My response, in most cases, has been blunt and to the point: "Brother, it's your penis. Therefore, it's your responsibility to cover it up." At its core, responsibility is the ability to respond to the consequences of your choices and actions. You do have the power to make choices. The only way to experience that power is to examine the options and the possible consequences, and then choose those actions that will create the outcome you desire.

Though anger and blame were the surface responses I got when I asked men about this issue, I detected an even stronger emotion running beneath: fear. I'm in no way making excuses for Garen or any other man who sires and then abandons a child. I do believe, however, that disempowerment has created a tremendous amount of fear in men. The fear of being wrong and then being criticized for it. The fear of losing and being abandoned. The fear of not doing something right and being shot down.

Fear is rooted in the belief that you're powerless. In contrast, being a father—producing life, re-creating yourself—is a powerful act. I can imagine that the biological act of fatherhood is well nigh overwhelming to a person who's been psychologically stripped of personal power. Some men probably truly believe that they can't stick around to be a father; the emotional risk is simply too great for them. Rather than allowing themselves to be shot down yet again, made to feel wrong or inadequate yet again, they abandon a piece of their spirit.

Until you believe that you have the power to make choices, you can't respond to the decisions you face with response-ability. And yet until you assume responsibility for your choices and actions, you can't experience a sense of personal power.

As a spiritual principle, responsibility is developed through the acknowledgment and acceptance of the presence of Spirit in your life and through practices that strengthen the sense of connection to Spirit. When you're consciously aware of Spirit, you receive guidance in making choices. As your choices and the consequences of them become clear to you, your ability to respond is enhanced.

Garen has to look into himself and see that fear has him by the throat. He has to realize that he reacts the only way he knows how when he's gripped by that fear: he abandons everything—his child, his child's mother, and himself. And each time he panics and runs, the fear gets bigger.

Fear is a powerful source of energy, if Garen can harness it. He needs to turn his fear into something that fuels good choices instead of flight. There are transformational power tools that will help Garen do just that, but they'll work only if and when he decides he's ready to choose his life rather than have his life choose him.

Transformation Plan and Power Tools

The three A's—awareness, acknowledgment, and acceptance—are Garen's primary power tools, along with the all-important responsibility. Garen's job is to go from his reaction-based, fear-filled, and powerless approach to life to an approach whereby he sees and assesses his options, chooses carefully, and carries out his choices with responsibility.

Choice is an important aspect of the spiritual reality. The dictionary defines choice, in its adjective form, as "worthy of being chosen; selected with care; of high quality." In its noun form it means "the *power* of selecting."

If you were told that you'd *chosen* to be broken and beat-up, you'd scream out your denial, but it's true. Though few men understand or believe in choice, no matter what's going on in your life, you always have the ability to make choices. In fact, the outward conditions of your life reflect the choices you've made (or failed to make).

What have you chosen to believe about yourself? What choices have you made based on those underlying beliefs?

What have you chosen to believe about other people and what they can do to you or prevent you from doing?

If you've believed little and chosen poorly, that can change. Through awareness and acceptance that Spirit, the presence of God, is active in your life, you can become more able to choose thoughts, words, and actions that reflect the belief that there's a power of good present in your soul.

How do you begin the process of moving from a physical to a spiritual sense of being? You begin by walking into your bathroom and standing before the mirror, looking yourself squarely in the eyes, and saying, "I love you." You begin by having genuine affection for yourself. Whether you're broke, unemployed, divorced, or all of the above, whether you're an ex-con or a corporate executive fearful of the glass ceiling, you're a child of the Most High.

But how do you love yourself when you're a man who feels unacknowledged, unappreciated, and angry at the world? How do you love yourself when you know that you've made mistakes but haven't yet admitted the specifics to yourself or anyone else? You may have left your wife for another woman, for example, and now you're about to leave *her*. You may have ignored your child's birthday because you didn't have the money for a gift. You may have ruined your credit buying things you really didn't need and *knew* you couldn't afford. You may drink a little (or a lot), snort a little (or a lot), and tell big lies to the people dearest to you. Given all that, how can you be at home with yourself? How can you see Spirit in your own humble spirit? How can you love the face you see in the mirror?

The same way God does: totally unconditionally, without reservation. God's Spirit within you realizes that you're growing through your experiences to that point where you'll become willing to become aware of and accept the presence of God in your soul as your source, your supply, your guidance, and your protection. When you finally accept that truth and that beneficence, you'll make better choices. And when you make better choices, you'll evolve from a limited human being to an enlightened spiritual being and an exceptional man!

Awareness

Sometimes it takes monumental or catastrophic events to get our attention. In order for Garen to become aware of his life, he has to sire three children. Three beautiful babies. This third is his wake-up call from the Divine: *Be aware!*

Wake up to your life! Wake up to your responsibilities! Wake up to the fact that you're not alone in this; the Divine is here to help!

If you're not willing to become aware, your knowledge and beliefs are limited to human perceptions. But perceptions are formed in response to experiences and the assimilation of information, both of which are clouded by emotions. Fear, anger, shame, and guilt are toxic emotions that cloud your ability to perceive the truth. The experiences you men have, the tainted information you receive about who and what you are, lessen your ability to perceive the truth, hinder your ability to perceive the presence of Spirit, and keep you from moving from the human to the spiritual realm. That's why men who believe that they're broke *remain* broken. Why men who believe that they're beaten *are* beaten. Garen believes that he can't take care of a child, so he can't take care of his lovely new daughter or her siblings.

When Garen looks himself in the eyes and sees the fear there, he'll realize that the fear has been making his decisions for him. If he looks with awareness, he'll see that Spirit is there too, offering another way to live. This awareness will enhance an internal drive that will awaken mental alertness and strengthen the spiritual connection with the divine energy of life.

Acknowledgment

Three kids, three different women, one man. What's the common factor here? This man can't run anymore from his fertility. He isn't fooling himself or anyone else when he denies his paternity. All he's doing when he turns from his responsibility is taking the plentiful energy of his fear and feeding it to the lie—and the lie rewards Garen by digging a deep, dark hole into which he can flush his soul.

Acknowledgment is a fairly small step in the vast scheme of things. You can acknowledge something and still do nothing about it if you want. If it's too hard for Garen to swallow everything at one time, all he has to do is say to himself and the child's mother, "Yes, that baby looks like me; she's beautiful, and she came from me." He can even add that it scares him silly to have created a life because he doesn't have the tools as a grown-up to deal with her.

No action so far; just acknowledgment. But even that sets up the whole picture differently: it allows decisions to be made—who will care for what; who won't. Even if what

Garen acknowledges is that he doesn't have the material, psychological, and emotional stuff to give this child and her mother, he still comes out ahead, because all that denial energy can be applied toward a solution instead of feeding the angry, hungry dog of fear.

Acknowledgment is key for Garen, because once he acknowledges his role in this child's birth, he is set up spiritually for responsibility. No acknowledgment, no responsibility. Yet this is what his soul craves: being responsible. Responsible for himself, for loving his children, for being a man in the world. Spirit says that we have to do our part. In denying our part, we deny the force of the Divine.

Acceptance

What a different energy gets created when we accept the things we can't change! Garen can't undo this child. She's there. Garen can't undo his fear either, unless he first accepts the fact that he's afraid, because acceptance is the key to personal power. Here he is, feeling helpless, powerless, and victimized. He feels that he has no choices. But he *does;* oh yes, he does.

Acceptance is an internal process. It's a psychological and emotional release of beliefs and thought patterns. Garen believes that he can't handle a child. If he can accept and then release that belief, he'll be able to see and deal with the fear that underlies it.

Because acceptance is the recognition of the power of truth and the presence of spiritual activity, it facilitates transformation. If Garen can achieve acceptance, it will give him that moment of psychological and emotional stillness he needs to subdue his fear, subdue his ego and its lies. Acceptance of his child's existence and of his own perceptions about parenting will create a shift in attitude and consciousness, and that shift will allow him to call on the Divine to help him with his fears and to help him take responsibility.

Responsibility

There's an affirmation I like that goes like this: *I'm responsible for the choices I make in life.* And that goes just as much for what I *don't* do as for what I *do.* In other words, failure to act is a choice.

Taking responsibility for his life, his actions, and his child will do exactly the *opposite* of what Garen fears: it will free him, not tie him down. All the energy that he's spent on running, denying, being angry and afraid will flow through him again the minute he steps up to the plate and affirms that he's responsible and will deal with the consequences. His fear and anger will dissolve.

Responsibility comes from a deep internal process, but it results in physical action. Based on the recognition of options and consequences, it results in conscious choice. Therefore, if you're responsible, you're powerful; if you're responsible, you're free. Nothing initiates personal empowerment more surely than responsibility. Nothing eliminates victimization faster. Nothing increases self-awareness more or honors one's personal strength better. Taking responsibility for what you do and for the results of your actions (or inactions) legitimizes your personal authority and increases your self-value.

Self-value is a huge part of responsibility, because when you love yourself, you can't walk out the door and walk away from your children. You know that they're a part of you, and you feel good about them as you do about you.

When you feel good about yourself, you make good choices about what you do, what you say, and how you conduct your life and affairs. This self-love, which is founded on the presence of God in your being and on God's Spirit moving in your life, gives you the patience and ability to trust that there's a rainbow on the far side of the storm. In other words, when you love yourself, you willingly surrender to the natural order and processes of life.

Garen was terrified that if he accepted responsibility for his child, he would have no more life. He would have to stay with the child's mother, and he might well mess things up with both of them. He linked responsibility with being a victim, with *having* to do something. Just the reverse is true. By claiming responsibility, he frees himself to actively make choices that create for him a role aligned with Spirit. No longer does he have to simply *react* to others' ideas of what his role should be.

As you become more responsible in life, it's important that you establish and maintain balance. Life is all about balance. You need to make clear, conscious choices that fill every moment of your life responsibly, taking full advantage of all opportunities available in all arenas. In Garen's case, for example, taking on fatherhood doesn't mean that he's *only* a father. It will mean that that is one part of who he is and he will only know that once he steps into the role, acknowledges his place in the natural order of things, and receives the power to perform his responsibilities.

When we take responsibility, when we align ourselves, in a balanced way, we receive the power from Spirit to do what has to be done as it has to be done, when it has to be done. We take our part, but it's *only* a part—one small part of a magnificent whole. Nothing will transform Garen's fear into power and freedom more quickly or completely than accepting responsibility for his actions and their consequences. In doing that, he takes his place in the natural order of things and receives the rewards of all that Spirit can offer in strength and self-love.

Knowledge Equals the Freedom to Choose

Freedom and choice are the keys to Garen's transformation. If he extends his hand to accept them, he'll go from being the victim of what his fear created to a man aware of his actions and empowered to do something about the world that his actions created.

Her face was etched into his mind. She reminded him of his sister. He remembered how his sister had cried about not having a father. He remembered the number of guys he had chased away from his sister, guys she had slept with. He remembered the number of times he had dragged her out of drug houses. He remembered the number of times she had called him because some guy she was sleeping with or running from had beaten her to within an inch of her life. He remembered the day he sat in court and heard the judge say, "Fifteen years to life." He remembered the last time he had visited his baby sister in the women's prison. That had been five years ago. He thought about her face and he wanted to cry, but he refused to.

8

Henry

Overcoming Feelings of Inadequacy

Henry realized that either he had lost his mind or he had taken talking to himself to a brand-new level. The voice was talking to him, but it was coming from within him. He turned the radio up. He could still hear it. He turned the shower on. The voice would not be silenced. Here you are! It's a damn shame! You turned fifty-five today and you still don't have your life together! Here you are, living in your sister's basement, again! Facing another birthday alone! Here you are, Henry! Now what are you going to do?

Henry took a deep breath and surveyed his current home. It was comfortable. It was clean. It was his refuge. It was his sister's basement. He realized that he had spent many years here on and off. It was the place he came to when he left a job, a wife, or a relationship. He wondered what he would have done, how he would have handled his life had his sister not had a basement. If he had no place to run to. No place to hide. Hey! I'm not running or hiding! Henry was talking back to the voice now. I'm just not putting up with crap! I'm going to be who I am! I'm going to do what I have to do! I'm just not going to take crap from anybody! Women give you a lot of crap and I'm not taking it! For a moment Henry believed he had silenced the annoying voice, but he knew he could not escape the feelings that the voice had unearthed.

Henry's story always unearthed feelings that he couldn't quite sort through. Henry had left college because his mother got sick and he wanted to help out at home. He worked two jobs to hold things together. He made sure everything and everyone was taken care of until his youngest brother graduated from high school. Then his mother died. She died without ever acknowledging Henry and all that he had done for his family. Henry couldn't quite sort that out.

After his mother had passed on, Henry's two younger brothers and his younger sister went to college. Henry thought about going back. It was a passing thought. Instead, Henry kept working to help his siblings. He eventually gave up his dream to go back to college. Instead, he fell in love and got married and kept working. He and his wife had two children. Henry bought the family a house. While he was working his wife stepped out on him. He was willing to forgive her, but before he could, she left him. Then she sued him for the house. After the court awarded her the house, Henry moved into his sister's basement for the first time. He went back to work, and every evening when he came home to the basement, he would have a few drinks just to help him get to sleep.

One of Henry's brother's went to law school; the other went into the Marines. Henry kept working. His sister also went to law school. Henry fell in love again, got married again, and had two more children. When Henry's sister graduated from law school, he was so proud he nearly burst. He wished that his parents had been alive to see it. He also wished they had been alive to thank him for all he had done for his brothers and sister. He settled for just feeling proud, since his sister and no one else seemed to remember all he had actually done.

Shortly after his sister graduated from law school, Henry's three-year-old son was killed in a car accident. It was then that Henry started drinking in the mornings. He had never stopped drinking in the evenings. He kept working, and he also kept seeing other women. It was the other women who encouraged Henry to leave his wife. It was his drinking that encouraged his wife to leave him. Henry's second wife took the second house. Even though he was still working, Henry ended up in his sister's basement again.

Many drinks, many jobs, and many women later, Henry decided to get himself together and finish his college education. He went into rehab, where he first heard the voice and first felt the pain and overwhelm of his feelings being unearthed. It was too much for Henry to handle. Although he followed his rehabilitation plan to the letter and learned a lot about himself, Henry never went deep enough into himself to get the answers he needed. Still, he emerged from rehab a changed man with a changed attitude.

Henry vowed he was never going to take care of anyone else. He promised himself that he would never lose himself or anything else to a woman. He decided that for all he had given and all he had lost, somebody owed him something. He wasn't quite sure who it was, but Henry vowed to get it!

When Henry's new attitude forced a supervisor to release him from a job, Henry retreated to his sister's basement. When his attempts to reunite with his first wife and then his second wife failed, Henry found himself back in his sister's basement. When Henry's girlfriends asked for too much or demanded a commitment, he retreated to his sister's basement.

On this night, his fifty-fifth birthday, standing in the shower of his sister's basement, Henry had the same overwhelming feelings he had encountered in rehab. He knew that somehow, somewhere, his life had gone horribly offtrack. It wasn't my fault! Sure he had made a few mistakes. But he had done the best he knew how to do. You think your father failed you! The voice was back. You think your mother abandoned you! You think your brothers and your sister are ungrateful! You think your wives were wrong! You think you've got it all figured out! The problem is you never gave yourself credit! You wanted it to come from everybody else!

Talking to the Man in the Mirror

When Henry looks in the mirror, he doesn't see anything. It's not that there's nothing there. It's just that Henry can't see it. He shut down his heart and mind so long ago that his vision has been seriously impaired.

Henry doesn't allow himself to think. He doesn't allow himself to feel. Beyond whatever it took to make sure that his hair was in place and that he didn't cut his throat while shaving, Henry simply didn't look at himself. In fact, he couldn't look. It was too painful, too frightening.

Henry had stopped looking at himself when his father died. He was afraid he would see the reflection of a murderer looking back at him. Henry had never told anyone that he felt responsible for his father's death. He avoided looking at himself when his mother died. He was afraid that he would see clear signs of her inadequacy etched into his face.

Henry had toyed with the idea of taking a deeper look at himself and into himself while he was in rehab. However, when he felt the truth rumbling in his soul, he thought he couldn't handle it. What difference would it make anyhow? He couldn't change what had happened.

Although Henry had decided to change his behavior and responses to his experiences, the changes took him further away from his true image. After his second divorce, Henry lost his desire to see himself or anyone else. He decided that not only would he shut out pain and people; he would push them away.

On the surface, Henry is a strong, attractive, able-bodied man with an insatiable appetite for women. He is a bit sullen, somewhat sad, and very complex. Right beneath the surface, Henry is a frightened six-year-old boy trying to win his father's approval and longing for his mother's nurturing. It's not that Henry is in any way inadequate. It's that he was never given adequate tools to deal with his very intense emotions. In other words, Henry is just like his father. He knows it, and he hates that about himself. He is also the spitting image of his mother. He also knows that, and it makes him furious.

Without the tools to deal with either of these realities, Henry chooses to hide himself in the three P's. He *protects* himself from further emotional injury or harm by shutting off his feelings. He *provides* himself with an escape route, alcohol, when his feelings are stirred. As long as Henry feels he can *please* a woman, which he seems to do pretty well, he can tell himself he is the best man he can be. Unfortunately, he no longer believes it.

My statement to Henry is, "Stop running! Stop hiding! Stop waiting!" Before I would say this to him, however, I would encourage him to cry.

Henry has fifty-five years of tears blocking his vision and his heart. For a man like Henry, I can imagine that crying is a difficult thing to do. If he allowed me to get close to him, I would cup his face in my hands, I would look him straight in the eyes, I would call upon the ancient mother of loving compassion and tender mercy who resides in my soul, and I would say, "Henry, you didn't do anything wrong."

I'm sure that he would squirm a bit, and he would probably

divert his eyes from mine. When that happened, I would move in closer, holding his face. I would kiss his forehead, connect with his eyes again, and repeat, "Henry, you are a good man, and you didn't do anything wrong."

Unless my mother instincts are totally off-track, that is all that would be needed to open the floodgates of Henry's pain. It is also all that would be needed to ignite his healing process.

There are moments in his life when all a man needs is the love of a mother. In those moments, any mother will do. If, in that moment, Henry would allow himself to be vulnerable, to hurt and feel his pain, to choose another story, to forgive himself for allowing himself to hurt for so long, his healing would begin. It is no coincidence that Henry's process began in the shower. Water is the universal symbol for the Mother.

Transformation Plan and Power Tools

Henry is about to get a lesson in self-acceptance, self-worth, and self-validation. It's not a lesson he wants; it's a lesson he needs! I've heard that men have three P's they believe they must fulfill in order to be men. They must provide, protect, and please. These P's drive a man. They give him a sense of value and worth. They give him something to do and a measurement for how he is doing.

In the process of successfully accomplishing the P's, a man needs support and encouragement. No matter how poorly or well a man does in his quest to provide for, protect, and please those he loves, without support and encouragement he feels as if he never quite measures up. He feels unsure of himself. He feels unappreciated and, in the worst-case scenario, inadequate. In Henry's case, as with many other men, there are many things a man can live with being and not being. Inadequate isn't one of them.

Life will give you every possible opportunity to change. It will also bring to you experiences designed to facilitate the inner and outer changes that will result in your personal growth and healing. In the face of the opportunity to change, in the midst of a life-changing experience, the choice to change is a matter of personal will. The will is a function of inner authority. It's a reflection of who you have decided you are and who you know yourself to be in response to your experiences, choices, and perceptions.

When you don't tell the truth or recognize the truth about your experiences. When you blame others. When you walk away and do not leave clean edges around your relationships or experiences. When you refuse to look at yourself or listen to yourself. When you make up stories about what really happened, and you believe the stories you make up, your experiences will become cloaked in dishonesty. That cloak will cloud and limit your ability to choose consciously. Consequently, your perceptions of yourself, your life, and what is really going on will be distorted.

A distorted self-image, supported by a distorted perception of reality, will hinder your ability to change. The only way through the distortions is to use your power tools. For Henry, the tools are willingness, forgiveness, acceptance, and choice.

Willingness

If you aren't willing to see the truth, you will never be able to see it. If you aren't willing to hear the truth, you will not hear it. If you believe your way, your thoughts, and your beliefs are right, no matter what anyone does or says, you will not move off your position.

Standing naked in the shower, Henry realized that he was going to see and hear some truth that he had been avoiding most of his life. For a split second, he became willing. That is all Spirit needs! One second of willingness can actually change your life if you're ready. Henry was ready to become willing.

Henry started out with three strikes against him that he had not been willing to investigate. First, he had a distorted perception of the man he modeled himself after. Henry perceived his father as a driven, raging, controlling, emotionally unavailable taskmaster. Henry perceived his father's harshness as a statement about Henry's inability to do things the right way.

It was the relationship with his father that planted the seeds of inadequacy in Henry's heart and mind. He had not been willing to consider that his father was a frightened man who was emotionally shut down in response to his own father's absence.

Instead, Henry made up a story about his father. Henry told himself the same story over and over. He told himself that his father didn't care about him and that he didn't love him. More important, he told himself that he would never be like his father. Eventually, Henry believed that what he was telling himself was true.

Henry was telling himself this story when his father had a heart attack, only moments after berating Henry for not doing something the right way. At his father's funeral, Henry began to tell himself another story. Henry told himself that if he had done the right thing, his father would not have had the heart attack.

The second strike against Henry was his mother's silence. Mom let Dad rule the roost, which is often the case when the man is controlling or raging. Henry told himself that women are weak because his mom had never stepped up to take a stand for her children in the midst of her husband's harshness. She never complimented Henry. She never supported him. She never encouraged him.

Henry needed someone, particularly his mother, to let him know that he was okay and that Dad was off the mark in some cases. Unfortunately, she never had the strength, energy, or courage to do it in the face of her husband's rage.

In Henry's mind the story went something like this: if you provide for a woman, she'll keep her mouth shut. She won't bother you. Henry never considered that his mother was as afraid of Dad as Henry was. He never considered that silence is not always a sign of weakness. In some cases, silence signals inner strength, the strength required to do what you believe needs to be done.

The third and final strike against Henry was his inability to ask questions and get answers, to look at himself and dare to feel good about what he saw, to do what was required or asked of him without the benefit of support or encouragement from the people who claimed to love him.

Henry's will had been challenged and damaged by his relationship with his father. His initiative never fully developed. In addition, Henry's heart, his emotional being, had been limited by his relationship with his mother. He never quite got over that because he needed to know that somebody was pleased with him.

Throughout his life, Henry had never taken the time to find himself, define himself, or accept himself. Instead, he focused his attention on the three P's, which is what his father had pounded in his head for the first fourteen years of his life. Henry did what he thought needed to be done for his mother, his siblings, and his wives because he thought he had to do it. Without their encouragement and support, without some report that he had done a good job, it had never dawned on him that he was also doing the things for himself. He was demonstrating his willingness to be of support and service to others.

Forgiveness

Henry didn't know that he needed to forgive his father. He didn't know why he needed to forgive his mother. He only knew that he couldn't forgive himself.

For most of us, forgiveness is a sensitive and very tricky

subject. On the one hand, we want to forgive and know we need to forgive. On the other hand, we believe that to forgive someone is somehow saying that what they did was okay. Forgiveness doesn't let the other person off the hook. It eliminates the hook altogether. Forgiveness is the only path to acceptance. Not until we can accept an experience without the judgmental story we often attach to it are we free to choose another way of seeing things.

Henry believed that his father knew what he was doing and that he didn't care how it affected others. After all, he was a man! Men provide, protect, and please. Men are deliberate and calculating. It never dawned on Henry that the face his father wore masked his own feelings of inadequacy. Instead, Henry chose to hold on to the anger, fear, and feelings of intimidation and inadequacy that were planted in his heart and mind as a young boy.

Henry didn't realize that his father didn't know any better. Henry didn't understand that the manhood tools his father had been given were inadequate. He used those tools in rearing Henry because they were all he had. For that he also needed to be forgiven.

Finally, Henry could not fathom in his mind that the last thing his father wanted to do was to hurt his son in any way.

Instead, Henry chose to make up and hold on to the story he told himself about his father. Henry couldn't see that it was the story and not his father that had caused his pain.

Forgiving his father would have opened Henry's eyes to a new level of understanding, understanding that although he didn't feel good about his relationship with his father, that relationship was the only one he would ever have. Henry had to learn to accept it for what it was and to be okay with it.

One of the most challenging and painful experiences in life is to hold anger in your heart against your mother. Henry made another choice. He chose instead to see his mother as weak and inadequate. In fact, he saw in his mother his own inadequacy about dealing with his father. He was very uncomfortable with those feelings and blamed her.

Because he saw his mother as weak, he couldn't figure out why he needed to forgive her. It was simply the way she was. He was absolutely correct. Henry didn't need to forgive his mother. He needed to forgive himself for making up a story about her. He needed to forgive himself for judging her as weak and inadequate.

Henry needed to forgive himself for believing that what he thought and felt about his mother was also true about him. In essence, we never forgive for the sake of others. We always forgive to open our own mind, eyes, ears, and hearts to the truth. The truth is people do what they do, which is the best they can. The truth is even when someone's best has a negative impact on you, you can choose how to respond.

Knowledge Equals the Freedom to Choose

It was becoming clear to Henry that he had made some pretty poor choices throughout his life. It was even clearer that those choices had been very costly to his self-image and sense of worth.

But what about the women? What about what they did? Am I responsible for what they did? What about my brothers and my sister, never so much as saying thank you? Always putting me down for not finishing school! What about that?

At every moment you are choosing what you see, what you hear, and how you respond. Henry had chosen to see the worst, hear the worst, and expect the worst. He had gotten exactly what he expected from himself and for himself. He chose the stories he told himself about himself and everyone else. He chose to leave school. He chose work over being present and active in his relationships. He chose to drink to mask his pain. He chose the women who left him. He chose to run and hide in his sister's basement. Henry chose to close his heart, to deny his feelings, to avoid dealing with things when they stirred within him feelings of inadequacy.

You can't escape yourself! You will show up in your life as other people, experiences, and situations that must be handled. How you handle or do not handle people, feelings, and experiences is always a matter of choice.

Epilogue

There are some questions that will come to mind as you begin or further your journey of transformation. How do I know if I am doing it right? That's your ego, tempting you to doubt yourself. There is no one way, one formula, one standardized approach to spiritual enlightenment. As a matter of fact, the worst experience of your life may be the very thing that turns you on to a deeper understanding.

What can I expect once I begin to live with these power tools in my life? Change. Everything will begin to change. How you feel, the way things look, how things sound will all change. Things that were once very important to you will no longer be that way. People you once thought were the cat's meow will not be able to get near your milk bowl. As you expand your consciousness, your understanding will evolve and everything around you will change. Keep in mind that no one is right, no one is wrong; everyone is uniquely divine.

In completing this work, I realized two things. The first is that this work is absolutely necessary. It is necessary because I have seen no concentrated effort beyond traditional religious communities to provide men with the process required for spiritual evolution and transformation. Spirituality is not anything that you do. It is what you are. You are that by divine right.

I also realize that this book is totally unnecessary because you do not need anything to get to that place of God within yourself. A book will not take you there. No lecture, seminar, or workshop will open that door. That place is in your heart. When you find it, you will transcend every experience, every tidbit of information, every thought you have ever had. When you find God right in the center of your being, it will literally blow your mind! All you need to transform and all you need to get to God is sincere desire and the expectation that you will get there.

Remember your emotions—the good, the bad, and the ugly—are God-given and they are the keys to your transformation. Use the energy these emotions give you to challenge yourself to reclaim the beautiful power and freedom that God intends for you. Remember that when you invite these tools, and when you invite Spirit, into your life, there will be good days and bad days. Remember to stay centered. There will be challenges that will force you to stretch and reach beyond your comfort zone. Trust the presence of God in you to protect and guide you. Throughout your process, carefully monitor your thoughts and emotions. When you find yourself thinking, feeling, or behaving in a way you know is old behavior, counterproductive, put yourself in check. When you start getting into chasing money, being famous, and showing other people what you can do, know that you are headed for trouble.

Use your tools. Do it differently.

As you begin to transform and grow, you will no longer confuse who you are with what you do. You will have the freedom you seek, and it will come from inside and your spirit will be lifted. Use your power to take you UP FROM HERE.

Acknowledgments

Words are simply ingredients to express the depth of my gratitude.

Liz Perle and the editorial staff of Harper San Francisco, I owe you big-time for this one!

Drs. Ron and Mary Hulnick, for being yourself and giving of yourself to the degree that you gave me the courage to be myself and to not apologize for it.

Norm L. Frye, for supporting me in moving beyond the self-imposed veil into the true light of Spirit with grace and ease.

Steve Hardison, coach extraordinaire, this one is for you and all that you have taught me about myself.

Acknowledgments

Ellsworth Chytka, my teacher and friend, you will always have a special place in my heart. As always, the staff of Inner Visions Institute for Spiritual Development, you are the living testimony that every prayer is always answered.

Rev. Michael Beckwith, Dr. Wayne Dyer, Dr. Deepak Chopra, and Dr. Bernie Siegel, for being such brilliant demonstrations of men living spirit-filled lives.

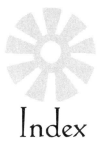

Index

accountability, 160
acknowledgment: benefits
    of, 53–54; described,
    52–53; Eddie's use of,
    123–24; Gabriel's use of,
    146–47; Garen's use of,
    187–88; Martin's use of,
    165–66; Phillip's use of,
    102. *See also* responsibility
acting out behavior, 88–90
African male rituals, 143
alcohol: fear dulled through,
    32–33; Henry's use of,
    196–97

anger: acting out due to,
    89–90; against mother,
    208; awareness of our,
    48–49; freedom to choose
    and, 68–71; key symptoms
    of, 38; power underneath
    the, 8; recognizing male,
    6–7; Roy's feelings of,
    39–40
authenticity, 26–27
awareness: Eddie's use of,
    121–22; Gabriel's use of,
    144–46; Garen's use of,
    185–87; Martin's use of,

awareness *(continued)*
164–65; Phillip's use of,
102; of Spirit, 50–51; spiritual mastery through,
51–52; of your emotions,
48–50

behavior: acknowledging
your own, 21; acting out,
88–90; conflicts between
self-beliefs and, 98–99;
examining and changing
our, 19–20; freedom to
choose, 67–71; seeking
pleasure/avoiding pain,
81, 82; silencing and bullying, 39; as symptoms of
emotions, 37–38; taking
responsibility for our,
63–65; taking right action,
66, 126; three Cs (control,
cooperate, compromise)
and, 71; value system of

society conditioning,
116–17
being (spiritual nature of),
3–4
beliefs: acceptance and emotional release of, 124–25;
conflicts between behavior and, 98–99; fear
founded on powerlessness, 181–82; power of
selecting, 183–84. *See also*
inner reality
blame: as distraction, 11;
Martin's use of, 160–61;
truth vs., 23–24
bullying behavior, 39

change. *See* transformation
process
clarity, 62
commitment: Phillip's use
of, 104–5; as spiritual
power tool, 62

communication/symbolic
    meanings, 78–79
confession: Martin's use of,
    166–67; as spiritual power
    tool, 56–58
confidence, 25–26
conscious breathing, 129–30
courage, 33
Creator. *See* God

desire to change, 44–45
discipline to maintain
    change, 45–46
distorted self-image, 202–3
drug testing, 33

E-g-o (Easing God Out), 10
Eddie: bad habits/problems
    facing, 112–20; behavior
    of, 108–12; knowledge/
    freedom to choose and,
    128–32; reclaiming spiri-
    tual core, 118–20; use of

transformation plan/
    power tools by, 121–28
ego: action triggered by,
    10–11; controlling
    demands of, 130; inner
    realities feeding, 91–93;
    speech motivated by, 79;
    subdued through still-
    ness/conscious breathing,
    129–30; surrender of
    the, 60
emotional charge, 83
emotional negotiation
    skills, 80
emotional reality, 83–84
emotions: behavior symp-
    toms of, 37–38; being
    blinded by our, 28; fed by
    inner reality, 90–93; free-
    dom to use power of,
    67–71; naming and claim-
    ing your, 11; surrendering
    to your, 59; transformation

emotions *(continued)*
through negative, 9,
212–13; understanding
negative/toxic, 7–8;
understanding transfor-
mation through, 18–19
energy: of emotions, 28;
sense of renewed, 24–25.
See also spiritual energy

fatherhood: abandonment of
children and, 180–81; taking responsibility for, 191
fear: ability to respond lessened by, 178–80; acting
out due to, 89; dulled
through alcohol, 32–33;
fed by inner reality, 91;
founded on powerless-
ness belief, 181–82;
power underneath the, 8;
recognizing men and
their, 6; responsibility

weakened by, 178. *See
also* terror
forgiveness: Henry's use of,
206–9; Martin's use of,
167–68; Phillip's use of,
103–4; as spiritual power
tool, 60–61; women's
assistance through, 7
freedom of thought/expres-
sion/movement, 84
freedom to choose: Eddie's
use of knowledge and,
128–32; Gabriel's use of
knowledge and, 149–52;
Garen's use of knowledge
and, 192–93; Henry's use
of knowledge and,
209–10; Martin's use of
knowledge and, 169–71;
Phillip's use of knowledge
and, 105–7; spiritual
power tools/knowledge
equal, 67–71

Gabriel: behavior of, 133–38; knowledge/freedom to choose and, 149–52; self-image/powerlessness of, 138–42; use of transformation plan/power tools by, 143–49

Garen: behavior of, 172–76; knowledge/freedom to choose and, 192–93; self-assessment by, 176–83; use of transformation plan/power tools by, 183–92

God: accepting presence in life by, 185; acknowledging connection to, 10; self-love founded on presence of, 190–91; spiritual mastery and connection to, 9; trusting in, 213

God's love, 2–3. *See also* love

guilt, 166

healing, 15. See also transformation process

Henry: behavior of, 194–98; knowledge/freedom to choose and, 209–10; self-assessment by, 198–201; use of transformation plan/power tools by, 201–9

inner reality: activating spiritual energy of, 93–101; creation of, 80; emotional reality and, 83–84; mental reality and, 82; physical reality and, 81, 85; thoughts/emotions fed by, 90–93. *See also* beliefs

inner spiritual reality: challenge to live from the, 105–6; described, 84–85

Jordan, Michael, 26

knowledge: Eddie's freedom to choose using, 128–32; freedom to choose equal to, 67–71; Gabriel's freedom to choose using, 149–52; Garen's freedom to choose using, 192–93; Henry's freedom to choose using, 209–10; Martin's freedom to choose using, 169–71; Phillip's freedom to choose using, 105–7; on spiritual mastery potential, 131

lack of worth, 119–20
language symbols, 78–79
love: application to wounded places, 15; defining, 15–16. *See also* God's love

male rituals (Africa), 143

male spirit, 16–18. *See also* Spirit
man in the mirror: Eddie's assessment of, 112–20; Gabriel's assessment of, 138–42; Garen's assessment of, 176–83; Henry's assessment of, 198–201; Martin's assessment of, 160–63; Phillip's assessment of, 85–90; Roy's assessment of, 34–41
Martin: knowledge/freedom to choose using, 169–71; self-assessment by, 160–63; stages of leaving behind of, 153–60; use of transformation plan/power tools by, 163–69
masculinity: sissy label and, 4–5; the spiritual essence of, 4; women's influence on models of, 149

men: African rituals celebrating manhood of, 143–44; brutality of personal experiences by, 17; children abandoned by, 180–81; defining what it means to be, 3–4; importance of God's love to, 2–3; recognizing fear in, 6; role of women in lives of, 6–7; taught what to do vs. be, 4–6; three Cs (control, cooperate, compromise) and, 71; three Ps (provide, protect, please) and, 201–2; value system of society conditioning, 116

mental reality: described, 82; Phillip's experience with, 85–90

mind-body communion, 25

Native Americans, 16

negative emotions: as secret to transformation, 9, 212–13; understanding, 7–8

pain avoiding behavior, 81, 82

Phillip: behavior of, 75–78; inner reality triggering behavior of, 92–93; knowledge/freedom to choose and, 105–7; physical and mental reality of, 85–90; spiritual energy activated by, 97–101; use of transformation plan/power tools by, 101–5

physical reality: described, 81; Phillip's experience with, 85–90

plan of Spirit, 150, 151

pleasure seeking behavior, 81, 82

polish the shell, 145

power: as born in darkness, 9; of freedom to choose, 67–71; responsibility as synonymous with, 62–63, 168–69; transformation and sense of true, 27; underneath negative emotions, 8

power of selecting, 183–84

powerlessness: fear founded on feelings of, 181–82; Gabriel's self-image and, 138–42

prayer, 7

reality. *See* inner reality

recognizing needed change, 44

relationships: emotional negotiation skills and, 80; surrender as essential to, 59; symbolic meanings of language and, 78–79

responsibility: for activating spiritual energy, 94–95; developed through Spirit, 182; Garen's use of, 189–92; Martin's use of, 165–66, 168–69; Phillip's use of, 103; process for taking, 63–65; as spiritual principle, 99–100, 182; as synonymous with power, 62–63, 168–69; weakened by fear, 178. *See also* acknowledgment

right action: described, 66; Eddie's path to, 126. *See also* behavior

role models: Eddie's lack of, 142; Roy's poor, 31

Roy: angry feelings of, 39–40; awareness tools

used by, 49–50; descrip-
tion of, 30–34; self-
destructive behavior of,
34–41; substance abuse by,
32–34, 35–36; tools for
achieving transformation,
41–67; willingness to feel
anger, 46–48

Self: conflicts between
behavior and beliefs
about, 98–99; distorted
image of, 202–3; transformation process and,
73–74
self-love, 190–91
self-respect, 126
self-value, 190
self-worth, 119–20
silencing behavior, 39
Spirit: describing essence
of, 5; invited into your
life, 213; plan of, 150,

151; purpose within your
life of, 6; recognizing the,
9; responsibility devel-
oped through, 182; still-
ness and accepting help
of, 67; understanding
beginning of, 61. *See also*
male spirit
*The Spirit of a Man: A Vision
of Transformation for Black
Men and the Women Who
Love Them* (Vanzant), 2
spiritual energy: activated by
Phillip, 97–101; changes
in male role and, 118; how
to activate, 94–95; principles for activating, 95–97.
See also energy
spiritual mastery: knowl-
edge on potential of, 131;
meaning of, 10, 129;
requirements of, 9; truth
as key to, 51

spiritual power tools: acceptance as, 54–55; acknowledgment as, 52–54; awareness as, 48–52; commitment as, 62; confession as, 56–58; described, 41–43; Eddie's use of, 121–28; forgiveness as, 60–61; freedom to choose through, 67–71; Gabriel's use of, 143–49; Garen's use of, 183–92; Henry's use of, 201–9; Martin's use of, 163–69; Phillip's use of, 101–5; responsibility as, 62–65; right action as, 66; stillness as, 67; surrender as, 58–60; understanding as, 61–62; willingness as, 43–48. *See also* transformation process

spiritual principles: accepting reality as key to, 125; activating spiritual energy using, 95–97; responsibility as, 99–100, 182

spiritual reality, 93–94, 183–84. *See also* inner spiritual reality

stillness: accepting help of Spirit and, 67; Eddie's search for, 126–28; to subdue ego, 129–30

substance abuse: by Henry, 196–97; by Roy, 32–34, 35–36

surrender: Martin's use of, 167; as spiritual power tool, 58–60

symbolic language, 78–79

terror: being brutalized through, 2; being controlled through, 1; limiting beliefs of, 17–18. *See also* fear

three Cs (control, cooperate, compromise), 71

three Ps (provide, protect, please), 201–2

toxic emotions. *See* negative emotions

transformation process: assessing your own, 211–12; as being about Self, 73–74; necessity of, 212; negative emotions as secret to, 9, 212–13; personal nature of, 14–15; promise of the, 24–29; truth and, 21–24; two things to ease the, 14; understanding role of emotions in, 18–19; walking gently on the earth and, 19–20; work involved in the, 8–9. *See also* spiritual power tools

truth: in acknowledging your behavior, 21–22; acknowledgment as recognition of, 52–53; as key to spiritual mastery, 51; through confession, 56–58; transformation and role of, 21–24; understanding revelation of, 61–62

understanding: Gabriel's use of, 147–49; negative/toxic emotions, 7–8; as spiritual power tool, 61–62; transformation through emotions, 18–19

walking gently on the earth: changing behavior to, 19–20; Native Americans philosophy on, 16

willingness: Henry's use of, 203–6; importance of,

willingness *(continued)*
43–44; three components
of, 44–46
women: influence on mas-
culinity models by, 149;
prayer and forgiveness of,
7; role in lives of men by,

6–7; value system of society conditioning, 116–17
wounded places: acting out
behavior due to, 88–90;
application of love to, 15;
looking at your, 14–15